Curing Chronic Fatigue Syndrome and Fibromyalgia with Paleo (Recipes Included)

by Lily Penrose

Table of Contents

- Introduction 6
  - Symptoms 6
  - When to see a doctor 7
  - Causes 7
  - Risk factors 7
  - Complications 8
  - Treatments and drugs 8
  - Therapy 9
  - Lifestyle and home remedies 9
  - Alternative medicine 10
  - Coping and support 10
  - How it affects quality of life 11
  - Different terms for the condition 11
- Paleo Diet 12
  - Building A Healthy Paleo Diet 12
  - Health Benefits of a Paleo Diet 13
  - Does it work for diabetes? 14
  - Cardio Vascular Disease 14
  - Autoimmunity 14
  - Guidelines 15
  - Treating chronic fatigue syndrome 17
  - Chronic Fatigue and Diet 17
  - Nutrients and Nutrient Deficiencies 18
  - Mental or Physiological Stress 18
  - Infections, Immunity, and Autoimmunity 19
  - Gut Health 19
  - Diet and CFS: What's the Evidence that it Actually Helps? 19
  - Keeping it All in Perspective 21
  - Causes of Chronic Fatigue Syndrome 21
- 4 Steps Towards Overcoming Chronic Fatigue Syndrome 22
  - Step 1: Eliminate Food Sensitivities and Allergens 22
  - Step 2: Increase Your Vitamin B Intake 24
  - Step 3: Increase Potassium and Magnesium Intake 26
  - Step 4: Build Peace and Relax 27
- Chronic Fatigue/Fibromyalgia is Classified as an Autoimmune Disease 31
- Enter the Paleo Diet for Fibromyalgia 38
- What to Expect from the Paleo Diet 40
  - Tweaking the Paleo Diet for Fibromyalgia 40
  - Glutathione Depletion and Fibromyalgia 41
  - The Methylation Cycle and Fibromyalgia 42
  - Chronic Fatigue in Fibromyalgia 42
  - "Leaky Gut" and Fibromyalgia 43
- Paleo Recipes 45
- Soup Recipes 45
  - Very Easy Extra Quick Tomato Soup 45
  - Tomato and Vegetable Soup 46
  - „Cream" Of Chicken Soup 47
  - Tomato and Basil Soup 48
  - Carrot and Coriander Soup 49

- Super-Fast Tomato Soup 50
- Spicy Carrot Soup 51
- Italian Bean and Vegetable Soup 52
- Quick Pea Soup 53

Lunch Recipes 54
- Onion, Pepper, and Pea Tortilla 54
- Huevos Rancheros in a Hurry 55
- Healthy Veggie Sizzle 56
- Home-Made Sausage Patties 57
- Vegetable Omelet 58
- Curried Eggs 59
- Egg "Pancakes" 60
- Bean Fry 61
- Hummus 62
- Devilled Eggs 63

Meat Recipes 64
- Beef Stew 64
- Banger Surprise 65
- Beef Burgers 66
- Beef Burgers 2 67
- Beef Curry Stir Fry 68
- Beef Goulash 69
- Braised Silverside (Beef) 70
- Pot Roast Brisket 71
- Lamb and Herb Burgers 73
- Meat and Egg Loaf 74
- Stuffed Peppers 75
- Kebabs 76
- Pork, Herb and Apple Burgers 77
- Meat Loaf 78
- Home-made Sausage Patties 79
- Tex Mex Chili with Chili Cream 80
- Lamb and Vegetable Curry 81
- Lamb Meat Balls/Burgers 82
- Chili Con Carne 83
- Moroccan Meatballs 84
- Sausage and Bean Pot 85
- Simple Pork Stir – Fry 86
- Sausage, Lamb and Pineapple Casserole 87
- Thai Beef Salad 88
- Easy Cassoulet 89
- Succulent Pork Chops 90

Chicken Recipes 91
- Thai Red Curry 91
- Chicken Kievs 92
- Spicy Chicken with Vegetable Sauce 93
- Ham, Chicken & Tarragon Pie 95
- Chicken Curry 97
- Oriental Chicken 99
- Moroccan Chicken 100
- Hawaiian Chicken 101
- Zesty Chicken Stir Fry 102
- Apricot and Nut-stuffed Chicken Breasts 103

3

Spiced Turkey Burgers with Guacamole Topping 104

Offal Recipes 105
    Liver, Bacon and Onions 105
    Beef and Kidney Stew 106
    Cod Ragout 107
    Quick Prawn Curry 108
    Seafood Curry 109
    Salmon with Herby Roasted Vegetables and Bacon 110
    Ginger and Spring Onion King Prawns 111
    Trout with Prawns 112
    Mediterranean Fish Roast 113
    Roasted Spiced Cod 114
    Tandoori Prawn Skewers 115
    Thai Steamed Salmon 116
    Fish Burgers 117
    Seared/Roasted Halibut 118
    Grilled Sesame Salmon with Rocket Salad 119

Vegetable Recipes 120
    Ratatouille 120
    Tomato Salsa 121
    Cauliflower with Tomatoes and Cumin 122
    Asparagus and Bacon Stir Fry 123
    Courgettes with Moroccan Spices 124
    Deep Fried Spinach 125
    Roasted Vegetables 126
    Sauerkraut 127
    Roasted Garlic and Lemon Cauliflower 128
    Courgette Pasta with Bacon 129
    Roasted Butternut Squash 130
    Oven Roast Cauliflower and Broccoli with Garlic 131
    Bean Filling for Stuffed Marrow, Courgette or Green Pepper 132
    Coleslaw 133
    Chickpea and Spinach Curry 134

Desserts and Puddings 135
    Easy Chocolate Mousse 135
    Chocolate Pudding 136
    Apple and Coconut Omelet 137
    Instant Hot Chocolate Almond Sponge Cake 138
    Faux Yo 139
    Stone Age "Ice Cream" 140
    I Can't Believe It's Not Ice Cream 141
    Chocolate Nut Torte 142
    Chocolate Mousse 144
    Raspberry Panna Cotta 146

Bread Substitute Recipes 148
    American Pancakes 148
    Savory Gram (Chick Pea) Flour Pancakes 149
    Yorkshire Oatcakes 150
    Wheat-free Rosemary-Thyme Crackers 151
    Flax Seed (Linseed) Loaf 152
    Low-carb Ground Almond Slice 153
    Broccoli Bread 154

Dressings 155
- Tomato Salsa 155
- Garlic Mayonnaise 156
- Lemon Vinaigrette 157
- French Dressing... 158
- Mayonnaise 159
- Sweet Mustard Salad Dressing 160
- Pesto 161

Milk Substitutes 162
- Double Cream 162

Snacks and Goodies 163
- Pork Scratchings 163
- Tapenade 164
- Cinnamon Swirl Cake 165
- Cinnamon Biscuits 166
- Chocolate Coconut Squares 167

Drinks.. 168
- Stone Age Coffee 168
- Bedtime Cocoa 169
- Stone Age Anytime Cuppasoup 170

Introduction

Chronic fatigue syndrome (CFS) is a complicated disorder characterized by extreme fatigue that can't be explained by any underlying medical condition. The fatigue may worsen with physical or mental activity, but doesn't improve with rest.

Chronic fatigue syndrome has also been called myalgic encephalomyelitis (ME) and, more recently, systemic exertion intolerance disease (SEID). Although CFS/ME and SEID share the same major symptom of chronic fatigue, there is variation between the definitions of these disorders. The symptom of chronic fatigue also may arise from more than one underlying condition.

The cause of chronic fatigue syndrome is unknown, although there are many theories — ranging from viral infections to psychological stress. Some experts believe chronic fatigue syndrome might be triggered by a combination of factors.

There's no single test to confirm a diagnosis of chronic fatigue syndrome. You may need a variety of medical tests to rule out other health problems that have similar symptoms. Treatment for chronic fatigue syndrome focuses on symptom relief.

Symptoms

Chronic fatigue syndrome has eight official signs and symptoms, plus the central symptom that gives the condition its name:

- Fatigue
- Loss of memory or concentration
- Sore throat
- Enlarged lymph nodes in your neck or armpits
- Unexplained muscle pain
- Pain that moves from one joint to another without swelling or redness
- Headache of a new type, pattern or severity

- Unrefreshing sleep
- Extreme exhaustion lasting more than 24 hours after physical or mental exercise

When to see a doctor

Fatigue can be a symptom of many illnesses, such as infections or psychological disorders. In general, see your doctor if you have persistent or excessive fatigue.

Causes

Scientists don't know exactly what causes chronic fatigue syndrome. It may be a combination of factors that affect people who were born with a predisposition for the disorder.

Some of the factors that have been studied include:

Viral infections. Because some people develop chronic fatigue syndrome after having a viral infection, researchers question whether some viruses might trigger the disorder.

Suspicious viruses include Epstein-Barr virus, human herpes virus 6 and mouse leukemia viruses. No conclusive link has yet been found.

Immune system problems. The immune systems of people who have chronic fatigue syndrome appear to be impaired slightly, but it's unclear if this impairment is enough to actually cause the disorder. Hormonal imbalances. People who have chronic fatigue syndrome also sometimes experience abnormal blood levels of hormones produced in the hypothalamus, pituitary glands or adrenal glands. But the significance of these abnormalities is still unknown.

Risk factors

Factors that may increase your risk of chronic fatigue syndrome include:

Age. Chronic fatigue syndrome can occur at any age, but it most commonly affects people in their 40s and 50s.

Sex. Women are diagnosed with chronic fatigue syndrome much more often than men, but it may be that women are simply more likely to report their symptoms to a doctor.

Stress. Difficulty managing stress may contribute to the development of chronic fatigue syndrome.

Complications

Possible complications of chronic fatigue syndrome include:

- Depression
- Social isolation
- Lifestyle restrictions
- Increased work absences

Treatments and drugs

Because chronic fatigue syndrome affects people in many different ways, your treatment will be tailored to your specific set of symptoms. Symptom relief may include certain medications:

Antidepressants. Many people who have chronic fatigue syndrome are also depressed. Treating your depression can make it easier for you to cope with the problems associated with chronic fatigue syndrome. Low doses of some antidepressants also can help improve sleep and relieve pain.

Sleeping pills. If home measures, such as avoiding caffeine, don't help you get better rest at night, your doctor might suggest trying prescription sleep aids.

Therapy

There's no known cure for chronic fatigue syndrome, and the most effective treatment for chronic fatigue syndrome remains uncertain. However, there's evidence that a multipronged approach may be helpful:

Pace yourself. Keep your activity on an even level. If you do too much on your good days, you may have more bad days.
Graded exercise. In order to improve daily function, more than pacing alone is needed. Previous studies suggest that graded exercise is an effective and safe treatment, but evidence for this remains limited.

A physical therapist can help determine what types of exercise are best for you. Inactive people often begin with range-of-motion and stretching exercises for just a few minutes a day. Slow, incremental increases in activity then take place over weeks to months.

If you're exhausted the next day, you're doing too much. Your strength and endurance will improve as you gradually increase the intensity of your exercise over time.

Psychological counseling. Talking with a counselor can help you figure out options to work around some of the limitations that chronic fatigue syndrome imposes on you. Feeling more in control of your life can improve your outlook dramatically. Cognitive behavioral therapy and self-management strategies are among the most helpful.
Not everyone who has severe chronic fatigue and post exertional malaise — intense exhaustion or mental fatigue after physical or mental activities that were once tolerated — responds to treatment in the same way. People who have a better chance of treatment success tend to have less impairment, focus less on symptoms, comply with counseling programs and pace themselves to avoid overexertion and under exertion.

Lifestyle and home remedies

For chronic fatigue syndrome, certain self-care measures may help:

Reduce stress. Develop a plan to avoid or limit overexertion and emotional stress. Allow yourself time each day to relax. That may mean learning how to say no without guilt.

Improve sleep habits. Go to bed and get up at the same time each day. Limit daytime napping and avoid caffeine, alcohol and nicotine. Pace yourself. Keep your activity on an even level. If you do too much on your good days, you may have more bad days.

Alternative medicine

Many alternative therapies have been promoted for chronic fatigue syndrome. It's difficult to determine whether these therapies actually work, partly because the symptoms of chronic fatigue syndrome often are linked to mood and can vary from day to day.

Pain associated with chronic fatigue syndrome may be helped by:

- Acupuncture
- Massage
- Yoga or tai chi

Coping and support

The experience of chronic fatigue syndrome varies from person to person. For many people, however, the symptoms are more bothersome early in the course of the illness and then gradually decrease. Emotional support and counseling may help you and your loved ones deal with the uncertainties and restrictions of chronic fatigue syndrome.

You may find it therapeutic to join a support group and meet other people with chronic fatigue syndrome. Support groups aren't for everyone, and you may find that a support group adds to your stress rather than relieves it. Experiment and use your own judgment to determine what's best for you.

How it affects quality of life

Most cases of CFS are mild or moderate, but up to one in four people with CFS have severe symptoms. These are defined as follows:

Mild – you're able to care for yourself, but may need days off work to rest.

Moderate – you may have reduced mobility, and your symptoms can vary; you may also have disturbed sleep patterns and need to sleep in the afternoon.

Severe – you're able to carry out minimal daily tasks, such as brushing your teeth, but have significantly reduced mobility, and may also have difficulty concentrating.

Different terms for the condition

Chronic Fatigue Syndrome – often used and preferred by doctors as there's little evidence of brain and spinal cord inflammation, which the term ME suggests; ME is also thought to be too specific to cover all the symptoms of the condition

Myalgic Encephalomyelitis (ME) – preferred by those who feel CFS is not specific enough and doesn't reflect the severity and different types of fatigue, and implies that fatigue is the only symptom (myalgic encephalopathy is sometimes also used)

Systemic Exertion Intolerance Disease (SEID) – a new term suggested in a 2015 report by the US Institute of Medicine, which implies that the condition affects many systems in the body (systemic); the word "disease" highlights the serious nature of the condition in some people.

Paleo Diet

The Paleo diet is the healthiest way you can eat because it is the ONLY nutritional approach that works with your genetics to help you stay lean, strong and energetic! Research in biology, biochemistry, Ophthalmology, Dermatology and many other disciplines indicate it is our modern diet, full of refined foods, trans fats and sugar, that is at the root of degenerative diseases such as obesity, cancer, diabetes, heart disease, Parkinson's, Alzheimer's, depression and infertility.

Building A Healthy Paleo Diet

Lean Proteins

Lean proteins support strong muscles, healthy bones and optimal immune function. Protein also makes you feel satisfied between meals.

Fruits and Vegetables

Fruits and vegetables are rich in antioxidants, vitamins, minerals and phytonutrients that have been shown to decrease the likelihood of developing a number of degenerative diseases including cancer, diabetes and neurological decline.

Healthy Fats from Nuts, Seeds, Avocados, Olive Oil, Fish Oil And Grass-Fed Meat

Scientific research and epidemiological studies show that diets rich in Monounsaturated and Omega-3 fats dramatically reduce the instances of obesity, cancer, diabetes, heart disease and cognitive decline.

Saturated fat has been demonized by our health authorities and media. What is the basis for this position on Saturated fat? Are current recommendations for VERY low saturated fat intake justified? How much saturated fat (and what types), if any should one eat? Without a historical and scientific perspective these questions can be nearly impossible to answer. Saturated fat consumption in ancestral human diets: implications for contemporary intakes.

One of the greatest deviations away from our ancestral diet is the amounts and types of fat found in modern grain feed animals vs. the amounts and types of fats found in grass fed or wild meat, fowl and fish. What we observe is wild meat is remarkably lean, and has relatively low amounts of saturated fats, while supplying significant amounts of beneficial omega-3 fats such as EPA and DHA. The take home message is that free range meat is far healthier than conventional meat: Fatty acid analysis of wild ruminant tissues: Evolutionary implications for reducing diet-related chronic disease.

Health Benefits of a Paleo Diet

For most people the fact the Paleo diet delivers the best results is all they need. Improved blood lipids, weight loss, and reduced pain from autoimmunity is proof enough. Many people however are not satisfied with blindly following any recommendations, be they nutrition or exercise related. Some folks like to know WHY they are doing something. Fortunately, the Paleo diet has stood not only the test of time, but also the rigors of scientific scrutiny.

With a very simple shift we not only remove the foods that are at odds with our health (grains, legumes, and dairy) but we also increase our intake of vitamins, minerals, and antioxidants.

Come on! Our Ancestors lived short, brutal lives! This Paleo Diet is all bunk, right?

The Paleo concept is new for most people and this newness can spark many questions. We like people to not only read about and educate themselves on this topic but also to "get in and do it." Experience is perhaps the best teacher and often cuts through any confusion surrounding this way of eating. Now, all that considered, there are still some common counter arguments to the Paleo diet that happen with sufficient frequency that a whole paper was written on it. Enjoy:

Evolutionary Health Promotion. A consideration of common counter-arguments.

Does it work for diabetes?

A great question to ask is "Does the Paleo diet work?" Here we have a head to head comparison between the Paleo diet and Mediterranean diet in insulin resistant Type 2 Diabetics. The results? The Paleo diet group REVERSED the signs and symptoms of insulin resistant, Type 2 diabetes. The Mediterranean diet showed little if any improvements. It is worth noting that the Mediterranean diet is generally held up by our government as "the diet to emulate" despite better alternatives. You can find an abstract and the complete paper here.

Cardio Vascular Disease

According to the CDC, cardiovascular disease is the number one cause of death in the United States. Interestingly however, our Paleolithic ancestors and contemporarily studied hunter-gatherers showed virtually no heart attack or stroke while eating ancestral diets. The references below will explore these facts to better help you understand the heart-healthy benefits of a Paleo diet.

Autoimmunity

Autoimmunity is a process in which our bodies' own immune system attacks "us." Normally the immune system protects us from bacterial, viral, and parasitic infections. The immune system identifies a foreign invader, attacks it, and ideally clears the infection. A good analogy for autoimmunity is the case of tissue rejection after organ donation. If someone requires a new heart, lung kidney or liver due to disease or injury, a donor organ may be an option. The first step in this process is trying to find a tissue "match". All of us have molecules in our tissues that our immune system uses to recognize self from non-self. If a donated organ is not close enough to the recipient in tissue type the immune system will attack and destroy the organ. In autoimmunity, a similar process occurs in that an individual's own tissue is confused as something foreign and the immune system attacks this "mislabeled" tissue. Common forms of autoimmunity include Multiple Sclerosis, Rheumatoid Arthritis, Lupus, and Vitiligo to name only a tiny fraction of autoimmune diseases. Elements of autoimmunity are likely at play in conditions as seemingly unrelated as Schizophrenia, infertility, and various forms of cancer.

Interestingly, all of these seemingly unrelated diseases share a common cause: damage to the intestinal lining which allows large, undigested food particles to make their way into the body. This is called "leaky gut and the autoimmune response".

Guidelines

A Paleo diet should be high in fat, moderate in animal protein and low to moderate in carbohydrates. Calorie counting is not encouraged, neither is portion control.

Eat generous amounts of saturated fats like coconut oil and butter or clarified butter. Beef tallow, lard and duck fat are also good, but only if they come from healthy and well-treated animals. Beef or lamb tallow is a better choice than lamb or duck fat. Olive, avocado and macadamia oil are also good fats to use in salads and to drizzle over food, but not for cooking.

Eat good amounts of animal protein. This includes red meat, poultry, pork, eggs, organs (liver, kidney, heart...), wild caught fish and shellfish. Don't be scared to eat the fatty cuts and all meals with proteins should contain fat as well. Learn to cook with bones in the form of stocks and broths.

Eat generous amounts of fresh or frozen vegetables either cooked or raw and served with fat. Starchy vegetables like sweet potatoes and yams are also great as a source of non-toxic carbohydrates.

Eat low to moderate amounts of fruits and nuts. Try to eat mostly fruits low in sugar and high in antioxidants like berries as well as nuts high in omega-3, low in omega-6 and low in total polyunsaturated fat like macadamia nuts. Consider cutting off fruits and nuts altogether if you have an autoimmune disease, digestive problems or are trying to lose weight faster.

Preferably choose pasture-raised and grass-fed meat from local, environmentally conscious farms. If not possible, choose lean cuts of meat and supplement your fat with coconut oil, butter or clarified butter. Also preferably choose organic, local and/or seasonal fruits and vegetables.

Cut out all cereal grains and legumes from your diet. This includes, but is not limited to, wheat, rye, barley, oats, corn, brown rice, soy, peanuts, kidney beans, pinto beans, navy beans and black eyed peas.

Cut out all vegetable, hydrogenated and partly-hydrogenated oils including, but not limited to, margarine, soybean oil, corn oil, peanut oil, canola oil, safflower oil and sunflower oil. Olive oil and avocado oil are fine, but don't cook with them, use them in salad dressings and to drizzle over food.

Eliminate added sugar, soft drinks, all packaged sweets and juices (including fruit juices). As a rule of thumb, if it's in a box, don't eat it. At the grocery store, visit primarily the meat, fish and produce sections.

Eliminate dairy products other than butter and maybe heavy cream. You don't need dairy, but if you can't live without it, read this article and consider raw, full-fat and/or fermented dairy.

Eat when you're hungry and don't stress if you skip a meal or even two. You don't have to eat three square meals a day, do what feels most natural.

Eliminate external stressors in your life as much as possible and sleep at least 8 hours per night. Try to wake up without an alarm and to go to bed when it gets dark.

Don't over-exercise, keep your training sessions short and intense and do them only a few times per week. Take some extra time off if you feel tired. Consider short and intense sprinting sessions instead of very long cardio sessions.

Consider supplementing with vitamin D and probiotics. Levels of magnesium, iodine and vitamin K2 should also be optimized. Iodine can be obtained from seaweeds. You probably don't need a multivitamin or other supplements.

Play in the sun, have fun, laugh, smile, relax, discover, travel, learn and enjoy life like a daring adventure!

Treating chronic fatigue syndrome

Treating CFS is incredibly challenging, and it seems like almost everything has been tried at one point or another: antidepressants, cognitive behavioral therapy, light boxes, you name it. But here's a look at some recent studies exploring a potential link between diet and CFS.

Chronic Fatigue and Diet

Nobody can find one "cause" of CFS in the same way that there's one "cause" of Chickenpox or strep throat. But there still are several suspected triggers, including…

- Nutrient deficiencies
- Acute stress (mental or physical)
- Infections and immune disorders (specifically, CFS often seems to show up immediately following an infection, such as mononucleosis or Lyme disease)
- Gut health and gut dysfunction

...and all of those potential triggers should sound familiar as problems that can be affected in various ways by diet and lifestyle.

Nutrients and Nutrient Deficiencies

Nutrient deficiency is probably the most obvious way that diet can modify any kind of disease. Specifically, for CFS:

- Vitamin D levels are lower than they are in the general population (although this could also be reverse causation: people don't get CFS because Vitamin D levels are low; their Vitamin D levels are low because they have CFS and tend to stay inside most of the time)
- Coenzyme Q10 (CoQ10) levels are also lower in people with CFS, and there's evidence that it may be causative. This study found that 69% of subjects who tried CoQ10 found it helpful
- Magnesium is another nutrient of interest. For example, a review found that magnesium supplementation was one of the complementary and alternative therapies with the strongest supporting evidence.

From a dietary perspective, here's how you could get more of those nutrients...

- Vitamin D: wild-caught cold-water fish, time in the sun, or a supplement if you can't get outside
- CoQ10: meat, organ meats, particularly heart, fish, and a little bit in vegetables
- Magnesium: nuts, spinach, avocado, most meat and fish

Mental or Physiological Stress

Stress also has a lot to do with diet and lifestyle. Even though we typically think of "stress" as emotional or psychological stress, food can absolutely contribute. Eating gut-irritating foods, or foods that you're personally intolerant to, is a physiological stressor. Omega-6

overload or a diet high in sugar can be an inflammatory stressor. And restricting fat, carbs, or calories counts as "stress," too!
This suggests that eating a low-stress diet might be helpful for CFS. Think anti-inflammatory foods, antioxidants, avoiding gut irritants, balancing Omega-6 and Omega-3 fats, and getting enough carbs, fat, and calories.

Infections, Immunity, and Autoimmunity

Then there's the question of infections and the immune system. There's mounting evidence that CFS has an autoimmune component. This is backed up by the fact that CFS is extremely common in people with Type 1 diabetes (an autoimmune disease), but it doesn't seem to be explained by blood sugar, and it's not so closely connected with Type 2.

Autoimmune diseases are definitely influenced by diet, so the autoimmune connection to CFS raises the possibility that an autoimmune diet might be an option to explore.

Gut Health

Finally, there's some interesting research connecting fatigue symptoms to overall gut health. In this study, for example, the researchers concluded that "the comorbid triad of IBS, chronic fatigue, and musculoskeletal pain is striking and may point to a common underlying cause." CFS also has significant overlap with depression and other psychiatric disorders, and considering that gut health is such a critical driver of brain health, the CFS-depression link is more evidence that some kind of gut problems may be involved. Since diet is so important in maintaining good gut health, this suggests that dietary therapies to improve gut function, like eating probiotic foods, might be part of a strategy for managing CFS.

Diet and CFS: What's the Evidence that it Actually Helps?

The research above implies that the ideal diet for managing CFS would be...

• High in important nutrients, especially magnesium, CoQ10, and Vitamin D.
• Anti-inflammatory and low in potential stressors.
• Designed to support good gut health and heal any problems that might exist.
• Potentially some kind of autoimmune-specific protocol.
• Not just a diet, but also a lifestyle including plenty of sleep and stress management.

So has any of this actually been tested? Actually, yes!

In a study, researchers found that all of their patients with CFS had problems with the mitochondria (these are the structures inside cells that provide energy to the cells). The researchers told 34 CFS patients to eat a diet that was essentially Paleo (which they entertainingly refer to as an "evolutionarily correct stone-age diet"). The patients were also instructed to take some basic supplements, get enough sleep, and manage their stress.

A Paleo diet would naturally be high in all the nutrients mentioned above, anti-inflammatory, and gut-healing, even if it wasn't specifically designed as an autoimmune protocol. Combined with the sleep and stress management, it basically hit all the important points. And just as you'd expect, all the patients who complied with the treatment protocol improved.

There's also some evidence that dietary antioxidants (which reduce oxidative stress and help fight inflammation) are helpful. This study, for example, found that chocolate rich in antioxidants helped improve chronic fatigue symptoms, but low-polyphenol chocolate didn't.
In other words, there is some evidence that Paleo-style dietary strategies can be one way to approach managing CFS.

Keeping it All in Perspective

With every article discussing something like "Paleo and chronic fatigue" there's the temptation to fall into the "miracle cure" trap. But if there is a "miracle cure" for CFS (unlikely), then we certainly haven't discovered it yet, and at any rate, food isn't it. CFS is a complex disease and eating more salmon or less sugar is not the "magic bullet" that will instantly erase such a complicated web of problems.

What food might be able to do is to help alleviate some of the stress, inflammation, and immune issues that precipitate CFS in the first place, or possibly help address those issues in people who already have CFS and are trying to manage symptoms so they can have a normal life. The human studies are still thin on the ground, but they do provide some evidence that a Paleo-style diet can help manage CFS if it's used prudently and in conjunction with treatment from an actual doctor.

Causes of Chronic Fatigue Syndrome

We still know very little about chronic fatigue, and sadly, the cause is still unknown. While researchers continue to search for the root cause of CFS, there are preliminary findings that hormonal imbalances, poor immune system response, viral infections, chronic low blood pressure and nutritional deficiency are contributing factors.

In addition, research indicates that chronic fatigue syndrome may be linked to oxidative stress, Celiac disease, and food sensitivities or food allergies.

Most researchers believe that it's a combination of factors that can vary from individual to individual. Viruses that can cause CFS include HHV-6, HTLV, Epstein-Barr, measles, coxsackie B, parovirus and cytomegalovirus.

4 Steps Towards Overcoming Chronic Fatigue Syndrome

Conventional treatment protocols treat the symptoms rather than the underlying causes. Often individuals with chronic fatigue syndrome are prescribed anti-depressants and sleeping pills. In many cases, the side effects from these drugs are actually worse than the original symptoms.

Instead, I recommend the addition of vitamin B Complex, alternative and complementary health practices, a well-balanced diet rich with potassium and magnesium, and the elimination of food allergens.

According to a study in the Journal of Alternative and Complementary Medicine, acupuncture, meditation, magnesium, l-carnitine and SAM-e (S-Adenosyl methionine), show the most promise in the treatment of chronic fatigue syndrome and fibromyalgia.

Step 1: Eliminate Food Sensitivities and Allergens

More and more research is pointing to a link between food allergies and sensitivities and chronic fatigue syndrome. Allergies to certain foods, pollen, metals and other environmental chemicals may be causing the rising number of individuals with CFS.

According to a study published in the Scandinavian Journal of Gastroenterology, IBS, fibromyalgia and chronic fatigue are linked, and researchers were surprised. In a study of 84 patients that had been referred for "unexplained digestive problems," nearly all patients (except for one) qualified for a diagnosis of IBS, 85 percent had chronic fatigue syndrome and 71 percent had fibromyalgia. The common denominator, researchers in this study believe, is poor digestion and food sensitivities.

Gluten & Other Common Intolerances

For example, one of today's most common food sensitivities is a gluten sensitivity. Lactose intolerance, a casein allergy and an intolerance of other common allergens also may be at the root of chronic fatigue. Other common allergens include tree nuts, peanuts, dairy, soy, shellfish and yeast.

I suggestion is to consider taking an IgG (Immunoglobulin G) test to help you determine the foods that you are sensitive to — then you can eliminate them from your diet. By getting rid of your personal known allergens, symptoms of IBS, ADHD, cystic fibrosis, rheumatoid arthritis and chronic fatigue can potentially be relieved.

Candida Imbalance

When ordering the IgG test, be sure to add on a Candida albicans test. According to a study published in the Journal of Orthomolecular Medicine, an astounding 83 percent of participants who followed an anti-candida diet experienced a reduction in their symptoms related to chronic fatigue syndrome!

My candida diet includes foods high in probiotics including kefir, yogurt, sauerkraut and kimchi, as well as green vegetables, flax and chia seeds, and unsweetened cranberry juice. It also requires the elimination of foods that feed the candida in the body. These include sugar, fruit, alcohol and grains.

When candida is left untreated, it causes an inflammatory immune response and creates holes in the intestinal lining, leading to leaky gut.

Casein

Casein, a protein in dairy, can cause serious allergic reactions. A casein allergy is more than just lactose sensitivity; it stems from the immune system producing antibodies to protect against protein and can cause the body to release histamine. This can cause hives, nasal congestion, wheezing, the swelling of the lips, mouth, tongue, face or throat, and even anaphylaxis.

Of course, the best way to avoid these symptoms is to avoid casein. This protein is concentrated in high-protein dairy products, including yogurt, milk, cheese and ice cream. However, most individuals will not have a problem with ghee or clarified butter.

H. Pylori

In addition, bacteria called H. pylori are believed to be a contributing factor, and they are common in nearly two-thirds of the world's population. This unfriendly bacterium attacks the lining of the stomach; left untreated, these germs can lead to stomach ulcers.

Researchers found that once H. pylori was out of the body of study participants, their physical and psychological symptoms, including those from IBS, fibromyalgia and chronic fatigue, got well.

Step 2: Increase Your Vitamin B Intake

According to a study published in the Journal of Royal Society of Medicine, researchers found a direct link between reduced vitamin B levels and chronic fatigue syndrome.

Vitamin B6

The study focused on B-6, riboflavin and thiamine, and researchers believe that B-6 (or pyridoxine) is particularly important. Vitamin B-6 rich foods include wild tuna and salmon, bananas, grass-fed beef, sweet potatoes, turkey, hazelnuts, garlic and cooked spinach.

Vitamin B-6 helps to prevent and relieve fatigue, and it supports a healthy immune system. As stated above, some researchers believe that certain viruses play a role in CFS, therefore increasing B-6 levels can be a helpful treatment. B-6 helps support T-cell functioning, allowing them to more adeptly fight infections.

Importance of Methylation

Methylation is the term given to the process in the body where methyl compounds (one carbon, three hydrogen atoms) are used in the critical functions of the body — immune function, energy production, mood, inflammation, nerve function, detoxification, and even DNA — all of which are challenges in chronic fatigue syndrome patients.

Methylation helps you process toxins, make hormones, and even helps in the production of neurotransmitters such as melatonin. How well your body can methylate effects all of these important areas. Poor methylation can lead to a variety of chronic conditions including certain types of cancer, cardiovascular disease, diabetes, allergies, digestive upset, mood and psychiatric disorders, and chronic fatigue.

Vitamin B12

Methylation requires Vitamin B6, folate and B12 in order to methylate and for your body to function at a cellular level. When you have a vitamin B12 deficiency, it impairs the methylation process and can cause numerous malfunctions that directly contribute to chronic fatigue syndrome.

It's estimated that nearly 40 percent of Americans have a vitamin B-12 deficiency. Many symptoms of the deficiency echo the symptoms of CFS. These include a lack of motivation, low energy, poor focus, poor memory, emotional mood swings, fatigue, muscle tension and more.

Vitamin B-12 can boost energy, reduce depression, prevent against neurological degeneration and protect against some types of cancers. B-12 is a critical nutrient that supports the methylation cycle and can help to stimulate improved moods, more energy and better cognitive function.

Vegans and vegetarians are at particular risk for B-12 deficiency, as it is most commonly found in animal foods. Vitamin B-12 rich foods include beef liver from grass-fed cows, sardines, tuna, raw cheese, cottage cheese, lamb, raw milk, eggs and wild salmon.

To effectively treat chronic fatigue syndrome, the B vitamins are essential. In addition to vitamin B–rich foods, a vitamin B complex supplement can help. Overall, the B vitamins work together to support healthy metabolic functioning, hormone production and vitality.

Step 3: Increase Potassium and Magnesium Intake

Research shows that both potassium and magnesium can help improve the symptoms associated with chronic fatigue syndrome.

Magnesium

In a study published in the UK medical journal The Lancet, chronic fatigue syndrome patients were found to have low magnesium levels that accounted for a low red blood cell count.

In this study, patients that were treated with magnesium supplements self-reported improved energy levels, a more balanced emotional state and less pain. At the end of the six-week study, all patients that were given magnesium had their red cell magnesium levels return to normal.

If you have chronic fatigue syndrome, consider adding these magnesium–rich foods to add to your diet: spinach, chard, pumpkin seeds, yogurt and kefir, almonds, black beans, avocados, figs, dark chocolate and bananas.

These delicious foods can help you overcome chronic fatigue, one of the symptoms of a magnesium deficiency, and support healthy nerve function, healthy blood sugar levels, blood pressure regulation, and much more. It's estimated that nearly 80 percent (!) of Americans are currently deficient in this essential mineral.

Potassium

Potassium is responsible for proper electrolyte balance in the body. Potassium-rich foods include avocados, spinach, sweet potatoes, coconut water, kefir and yogurt, white beans, bananas, acorn squash, dried apricots and mushrooms.

Symptoms of a potassium deficiency include the common CFS symptoms: fatigue, irritability and muscle cramps. Eating a diet rich in potassium can help to relieve these symptoms, particularly when foods that because allergies have been removed.

Step 4: Build Peace and Relax

CFS can be debilitating both physically and mentally. Suffering from persistent exhaustion, reduced brain cognition, chronic muscle and joint pain, stress, and even guilt takes a toll on the body, and psyche.

Long-term stress control and relaxation must be a vital portion of any protocol used to overcome chronic fatigue syndrome. While seemingly impossible, it's imperative that sufferers of CFS do their best to effectively manage stress, and rest.

The Power of Rest

"Rest" means more than just sleep. Dedicate one day per week when you don't have any responsibilities or commitments. Truly commit to a full day of rest. This gives your body and mind a much-needed respite — helping to fight stress, anxiety and exhaustion. It's also important during the week, if you are having a particularly difficult day, to not overtax yourself.

While regular exercise supports wellness and helps to diminish stress, individuals with chronic fatigue syndrome need to exercise at a controlled intensity. High-intensity workouts can leave you drained for several days.

Exercise Therapy

Exercise therapy has been shown to help with fatigue, mental clarity and depression in patients with chronic fatigue syndrome. According to a study released in the European Journal of Clinical Investigation, individuals with CFS were recommended to perform aerobic activities, at the clinic twice per month, in combination with at-home exercises for roughly 5-15 minutes in duration, five days per week.

Sleep

Chronic fatigue syndrome sufferers commonly experience difficulty with their sleep. In particular, falling and staying asleep, restless legs, nighttime muscle spasms, and vivid (sometimes frightening) dreams. It's important to establish a regular bedtime routine, which includes a physical and emotional wind-down period.

Yes, this means unplugging from technology —including computers, tablets, television, and smartphones — at least 90 minutes prior to bed. According to a recent study in the Journal of Clinical Sleep Medicine, the use of interactive technology devices one hour prior to bedtime results in poor sleep and general sleep disturbances.

Make your bedroom a haven for relaxation and escape from the stressors of the day. Your bedroom should be cool in the evenings to help facilitate sleep, and the lighting shouldn't be too harsh. Setting the stage for restful sleep really is half the battle to fall asleep fast and stay asleep.

Essential oils are wonderful to help when you can't sleep. Try a few drops in a diffuser or dotted on your temples. Essential oils that aid in relaxation and sleep include eucalyptus, lavender, valerian, Roman Chamomile, marjoram, bergamot, clary sage, jasmine and ylang ylang.

Avoid Stimulants

Avoid caffeine, alcohol and tobacco, as these stimulants can cause additional restlessness at night. Be sure to exercise at least four hours before going to bed, as exercise can also act as a stimulant and create restless sleep.

Relaxation Techniques

Incorporate deep breathing exercises, massage therapy, meditation, yoga and muscle relaxation techniques into your daily routine as they can help manage symptoms of chronic fatigue syndrome. As part of your wind-down routine, especially if you experience restless legs or muscle cramps at night, try massaging my homemade muscle rub into your legs, or take a nice relaxing bath with Epsom salts to soothe achy muscles.

Try progressive muscle relaxation during your wind-down period. The goal is to isolate each muscle group, and then tense and relax them. You can start at your head or toes, but many find that working the way up the body is more beneficial.

Start by visualizing the muscles in the target area, and then tense/contract them for five seconds; then relax and exhale through your mouth. Move to the next muscle group, tense/contract them, and then relax. Continue until you've completed each muscle group in turn.

This can help facilitate muscle relaxation throughout the body and encourage a good night's sleep. This process is also great during the night if you awaken to muscle cramps or restless legs.

Vacation Time

Take a vacation! A change of scenery is important from time to time, for it allows our body and our minds to recover from our daily lives. Get away with family or friends, or even by yourself, to fight burn out, relieve stress and stimulate closer relationships.

Travelling opens up new doors, changes our perspective, and gives our minds something to focus on instead of our daily tasks. Just like regular exercise, regular vacations and getaways are imperative for long-term health and wellness.

Ideas for soothing retreats include yoga weekends, trips to a dude ranch, a cottage on a quiet beach or lake, or a cabin in the mountains, with a stack of your favorite books.

Social Support

Chronic fatigue syndrome can cause a division in relationships, as sometimes people simply do not understand your level of exhaustion, pain, and lack of interest.

After you have eliminated foods from your diet that are causing the symptoms of CFS, and you've increased your Vitamin B, potassium and magnesium intake, your energy levels will increase.

Then reach out to your friends and schedule get-togethers where you can catch up, share a good laugh or two, and re-engage. Research has proven that social support is essential for maintaining psychological and physical health!

Chronic Fatigue/Fibromyalgia is Classified as an Autoimmune Disease

When I first started practicing, the medical community did not recognize chronic fatigue. They told patients, it's all in your head. As nutritionists/chiropractors, of course we helped patients with adjustments and good nutrition and helped them realize they were not crazy. Now, not only is the syndrome and all its corresponding symptoms recognized, it has been reclassified as an autoimmune disease!

Also known as Myalgic Encephalomyelitis (ME)/Chronic Fatigue Syndrome (CFS), as well as Chronic Fatigue Immune Dysfunction Syndrome (CFIDS), there have been recommendations for yet another name change to Systemic Exertion Intolerance Disease (SEID), with better established diagnostic criteria, by the Institute of Medicine in a report in 2015.

What is Myalgic Encephalomyelitis (ME)/Chronic Fatigue Syndrome (CFS)?

It is a compilation of various symptoms commonly reported as post-exertional malaise (PEM), unrefreshing sleep, concentration problems and muscle pain that typically lasts at least six months. Most folks with this problem have it for years.

Back in the early 2000's it wasn't taken seriously and patients found themselves going from one doctor to another trying to find answers.

Patients complained of unrelenting fatigue especially after any kind of activity. There was also the pain – unrelenting muscle pain in various parts of the body. I remember one patient who had MRIs of every part of his body trying to find out where the pain was coming from.

Sadly, they missed the key area of origin – the immune system and the brain. Back then we didn't have the scanning technology we have today.

Thankfully today we have evidence that this disorder is not all in the head at all.

Well, it is a little.

Structural Differences in the Brain in Myalgic Encephalomyelitis (ME)/Chronic Fatigue Syndrome (CFS)

A study published in the journal Radiology, found structural abnormalities in the brains of people with CFS using MRI scans. The imaging showed several crucial differences in the brains of the CFS and control participants.

People with CFS had a slightly lower volume of white matter, which connects regions of gray matter in the brain. They also had very high fractional anisotropy (FA) values, a measurement of water diffusion, in a specific white matter tract of the brain called the right arcuate fasciculus.

Another abnormality appeared in the cortex – an area of the brain that connects to the right arcuate fasciculus. In CFS patients the cortex was thicker than in the brains of the control participants.

According to the researchers, these structural differences could indicate brain inflammation.

Myalgic Encephalomyelitis (ME)/Chronic Fatigue Syndrome (CFS) is an Immune Disease

Researchers at Columbia University's Mailman School of Public Health have found that ME is a physical disease that may be triggered by an infection and in susceptible people, linger on as a hyper-stimulated immune response and become autoimmune.

This study, published in the journal Science Advances, involved analyzing the blood plasma samples of 298 CFS patients and 348 people without the disease.

The researchers found distinct physical biomarkers in the immune system of those with the disease. The researchers also found differences in those who have had the disease for less than three years and those who have had it more than three years.

Those who had the disease for less than three years had higher amounts of different types of inflammatory cytokines such as interleukin-17A.

High levels of interleukin-17A are associated with many chronic inflammatory conditions, such as multiple sclerosis, psoriasis, and rheumatoid arthritis.

These seemingly unrelated diseases – neurological, skin and joint diseases are in fact all autoimmune. Autoimmunity is really one disease process, but may be expressed in many different tissues and systems in the body.

People with autoimmunity commonly complain about chronic fatigue. With these study results we are able to connect the dots and help people more completely.

Big Pharma is jumping on these discoveries with more biologic treatments. These biologic drugs may help some folks but have some pretty serious side effects and are very costly.

These two important studies have brought us much further along in our understanding of ME and CFS. Now that it is classified as an autoimmune disease we can forge ahead with natural treatments that can help turn down the inflammation.

Natural Treatments for Autoimmunity Based in the 4R Approach

- Remove – gluten, dairy, egg, nuts and other potential allergens, as well as aspirin, NSAIDS
- Replace – support function in the digestive tract with enzymes and HCl if needed
- Reinoculate – the bowel with prebiotics and probiotics and a diet that includes resistant starch
- Repair – the gut mucosa with gelatin rich bone broths, L-glutamine and other nutrients

This approach attempts to uncover the actual cause and imbalances in each individual rather than simply putting a band aid on the symptoms. Each individual has their own set of imbalances and this needs to be corrected in a specific and individual way. Using conventional medicines that suppress the symptoms may be necessary alongside the integrative functional approach while healing is going on.

More and more there are chiropractors, naturopaths and functional medicine doctors that take this approach. As always, never change your diet, medicines or supplements without involving your health care provider.

One diet that has become extremely popular as a means to lose weight and combat certain health conditions is the paleo diet. You may have heard about this popular diet but you may be unaware of what it entails. The paleo diet is based on principles regarding the way cavemen ate many years ago. Cavemen didn't have access to sugar, high carb foods, grains and processed meals and snacks. Due to the fact that cavemen didn't consume these foods, they were a lot leaner and had fewer health conditions.

Recent studies have proved that adapting to a paleo lifestyle can calm the symptoms of CFS/ME and even encourage it to go into remission. Since the immune system is involved in this illness, the paleo diet has the ability to help in a number of ways. First of all, many people with chronic fatigue syndrome suffer from one or more nutritional deficiency. Since the paleo diet consists of plenty of fruits, vegetables, nuts, seeds, and lean meat, consuming high amounts of these foods can reverse deficiencies, and therefore improve symptoms.

Another way that the paleo diet can relieve symptoms of chronic fatigue syndrome is by strengthening the liver. By avoiding grains, sugar and processed foods, the liver has a chance to rest and rejuvenate itself. Since the liver is one of the most important organs in the body, as it must filter out toxins in addition to much more, the healthier the liver is, the greater its chances of helping to combat chronic fatigue syndrome.

In addition, a healthier paleo diet increases a person's consumption of antioxidants. Antioxidants are powerful and can fight free radicals in the body by encouraging regeneration of the mitochondria of the body's cells. This can help people to recover from chronic fatigue syndrome and many other illnesses. The process is usually gradual, and people will often see noticeable improvement in symptoms after a few months.

The paleo diet is a possible treatment option for people suffering from CFS/ME. Despite the massive amount of research on CFS/ME, there is no definitive treatment method. Doctors will often provide treatment based on symptoms, yet patients often continue to suffer despite trying various treatment methods. There is no guarantee that the paleo diet will reverse the symptoms of CFS/ME, but for many people, it has proved to be quite promising.

Although there is no conclusive clinical evidence to support its implementation, the Paleo diet appears to be a clear starting point and possibly the best diet for fibromyalgia. Favorable case studies are being reported by doctors.

Fibromyalgia is one of the most complex and misunderstood chronic diseases there is. With over thirty-nine serious symptoms identified as a part of the fibromyalgia syndrome picture, it is no surprise that the medical community has no cure for it.

However, anecdotal evidence is mounting in support of a modified Paleo Diet for fibromyalgia as the foundation of a treatment protocol for the disease.

The pain involved in fibromyalgia is due to a dysfunction in the central nervous system.

Irritable Bowel Syndrome (IBS) is associated in over 80% of fibromyalgia patients.

Standard prescription opiates only reduce pain by about 50% in a mere 30% of people with this disease. Many people with fibromyalgia become addicted to prescription pain killers.

Most fibromyalgia patients can point to a specific traumatic experience which triggered the onset of fibromyalgia.

Patients with fibromyalgia report daily pain levels between 5:10 to 9:10 on a standard pain scale, with zero being no pain and ten being the worst pain ever experienced in a person's life.

Besides chronic muscle and joint pain all over the body, fibromyalgia patients have difficulty sleeping, chronic fatigue, abdominal cramping, chemical, food, and environmental allergies, sinus issues, chronic diarrhea, mood swings, and chronic depression.

Any physical activity, even light housework, can trigger such incapacitating pain that employment and relationships become difficult to maintain.

Fibromyalgia patients often take prescription Cymbalta for depression and pain, the anti- seizure medication Lyrica, and trazadone or some other "sleeping pill."

They may take Lomotil for diarrhea, Requip for restless leg syndrome, Norco or even morphine for chronic pain, and Synthroid for low thyroid levels. Females often take prescription hormones.

Other medications may be taken to relieve the side effects associated with these prescription drugs.

Cymbalta, alone, though somewhat effective for fibromyalgia pain, causes weight gain, drowsiness, and a host of side effects associated with antidepressants. It is also expensive.

Enter the Paleo Diet for Fibromyalgia

The Paleo, Caveman, and ancestral diets are basically all the same. The foundational foods that make up the Paleo diet are grass fed and fatty meat, bone broths and soups, fermented foods such as sauerkraut or kimchi, and loads of vegetables.

All gluten is eliminated, along with most grains, and certainly, all junk and fast foods. Dairy is eliminated for the most part. Nightshade vegetables, including tomatoes, eggplant, peppers, and potatoes, seem to give many people with fibromyalgia trouble.

Also included in the "diet" is plenty of sunshine without sunscreen and exercise.

Body work or massage therapy, yoga and meditation, etc., are other alternative treatments for fibromyalgia which have been found to relieve symptoms of the disease.

It must be stressed that the Paleo diet is the starting point for people with fibromyalgia. It is recommended that the fibromyalgia patient stay on a strict Whole 30 or similar diet for a full thirty days, or even three months before making any further changes to the diet.

Some symptoms may be completely erased with the Paleo diet. Others will require a sort of "reverse elimination diet," where a food is added back, and reactions are noted over a week's time before adding a new food.

In this way, the fibromyalgia patient gets an idea of which foods trigger fibromyalgia symptoms and which are safe to eat.

In addition to the food portion of the Paleo Diet, many people with fibromyalgia are finding relief by taking a magnesium supplement. This can be magnesium malate, magnesium citrate, or magnesium sulfate, which is nothing more than Epsom salt.

Magnesium citrate and magnesium sulfate have a laxative effect. For fibromyalgia sufferers with leaky gut or irritable bowel syndrome, magnesium malate may be best tolerated.

Fibromyalgia patients are noticing relief from some of their symptoms by adding iodine to their diets in the form of either kelp or potassium iodide drops, selenium from eating two or three raw Brazil nuts daily, copper, and as much as 7,000 IU Vitamin D3 daily.

Fibromyalgia patients who have been on the Paleo Diet for any length of time are reporting:

- Candida albicans symptoms reduced
- Thyroid and upper respiratory issues reduced
- Insulin levels balanced
- More energy and less fatigue
- Less leg pain, joint pain, and body aches
- Environmental allergies and brain fog gone or reduced
- Desired weight loss
- Able to get off prescription drugs

What to Expect from the Paleo Diet

People who are using the Paleo diet to treat or overcome fibromyalgia report that it is a long process of tapering off drugs and detoxing from multiple food addictions. It may take as much as two months for symptoms to subside.

The key, according to anecdotal evidence, is to be consistent with the Paleo diet.

For a while, the fibromyalgia patient may feel worse. On top of the fibromyalgia symptoms come new symptoms from drug withdrawal and detoxification. Keeping a positive attitude while the body eliminates potentially decades of toxins is paramount.

Even within the Paleo diet, the fibromyalgia patient will need to customize the food plan. Food sensitivities are very individual.

One person may be able to eat coconut and coconut oil, while another person may not. Some can eat grass fed beef, while others must restrict their protein sources to sardines, salmon, and eggs.

Organic fruits and sweet vegetables like carrots help curb sugar cravings in the beginning stages. Berries, apples, bananas, and citrus are particularly helpful without throwing blood sugar levels off.

Fruit smoothies made with almond milk are an excellent way to get both complex carbohydrates and protein in the same meal. Raw nuts and seeds, as well as no sugar trail mixes can help to replace chips and popcorn.

Tweaking the Paleo Diet for Fibromyalgia

Tyramines can cause the blood pressure to rise, sweating, nausea, and migraines. Histamine can cause migraines, as well.

Most foods with tyramines and histamines are fermented: cheese, sauerkraut, yogurt, kefir, alcohol, kim chi, and vinegar. Fermented foods are encouraged on the Paleo diet, but if they trigger migraines, the person with fibromyalgia must eliminate them.

Arginine is a vasodilator. It opens the blood vessels, which lowers blood pressure. The only arginine rich foods allowed on the Paleo diet are nuts and dark chocolate. However, dilated blood vessels in the head can trigger a migraine.

Glutathione Depletion and Fibromyalgia

Glutathione may be the most important antioxidant in the human body. If the body has enough glutathione, it is well protected from oxidative stress and cell necrosis. If the body is low on glutathione, it becomes compromised and is at risk for all kinds of diseases.

Glutathione is the combination of glutamate, cysteine, and glycine. It is found in every cell in the human body. Glutathione determines how well protected we are from free radical damage from oxidation.

Not only does glutathione protect the body from free radical damage, it also helps with liver detoxification. It helps boost and balance the immune system to help fight off infections.

For fibromyalgia patients, it is important to note that glutathione also protects Vitamin B 12. Without glutathione, Vitamin B 12 is rendered inactive.

A blood test will not reveal a Vitamin B 12 deficiency in fibromyalgia, because the B 12 is there. However, a deficiency in glutathione causes Vitamin B12 to lose its ability to function in the body.

Anything which disturbs homeostasis, the state of optimal health, will destroy glutathione. This can be stress, emotions, bad food, environmental toxins, illness, pharmaceuticals, or a chronic lack of sleep.

The Methylation Cycle and Fibromyalgia

The methylation cycle causes chemical reactions in the body which make the amino acid carnitine, CoQ10, melatonin and other substances which are needed for neurotransmitters. The methylation cycle also controls sulfur metabolism and helps build new DNA.

On the DNA front, the methylation cycle helps to either prevent or silence gene expression. When genes are either over- or under-expressed, the epigenetics change in the cellular environment, which cause the symptoms of many complicated diseases.

Vitamin B 12 actually plays a critical role in the methylation cycle. In a fairly complicated chain reaction, Vitamin B 12 prevents inflammatory diseases, heart disease, and oxidative stress. It also helps in the production of cellular energy, or ATP.

Chronic Fatigue in Fibromyalgia

Chronic stress depletes glutathione. Glutathione deficiency leads to oxidative stress. Oxidative stress makes the body not be able to get rid of toxins fast enough, so they accumulate. Toxins cause the body not to be able to metabolize Vitamin B 12.

A lack of functioning Vitamin B 12 blocks the methylation cycle. A blocked methylation cycle causes sulfur not to be metabolized. Sulfur malfunction causes glutathione to become depleted, because sulfur helps to create glutathione.

This continuous downward cycle is why fatigue is chronic in fibromyalgia patients. Research is being conducted currently which addresses this aspect of the fibromyalgia picture.

"Leaky Gut" and Fibromyalgia

Along with chronic fatigue and misfiring pain receptors in the brain, fibromyalgia patients also have to deal with Irritable Bowel Syndrome, also known as "leaky gut," and the Gut and Psychology Syndrome (GAPS).

This breakdown in intestinal function leads to chronic inflammation in the entire body.

When the intestines "leak" toxins into the bloodstream and surrounding organs in the abdomen, it can cause liver damage.

When the liver is damaged, any number of the body's mineral reserves can become depleted. This degeneration happens slowly, over the course of several years.

Because fibromyalgia is so complex, it is a "syndrome" which is difficult to reverse.

Even with the promising results with the Paleo diet and treatment with magnesium, glutathione and Vitamin B 12, relief from symptoms and weaning from prescription pain medication and antidepressants is slow.

Patients who decide to try the Paleo diet for fibromyalgia should commit to the protocol for at least six months.

Adrenal Fatigue, Fibromyalgia, and the Paleo Diet

Once fibromyalgia patients do start to get more energy and see results on the Paleo diet, it is important for them to pace themselves.

Robb Wolfe and others who coach people on the Paleo diet state that many people who have adrenal fatigue and other illnesses push themselves too fast once they start feeling better. This causes a relapse.

People blame the Paleo diet for "not working," when the problem was, in fact, that the patients were overdoing it while they were still in healing mode.

Fibromyalgia patients must understand that any type of stress, including exercise, depletes the body of glutathione. Compromised individuals, such as those with fibromyalgia, will "crash and burn" if they try to do too much too fast.

Where Does the Fibromyalgia Patient Start with the Paleo Diet?

He recommends adding bone broths to this, and keeping the carbohydrate levels below 100 grams per day.

Certain starches are allowed during the beginning phase. These include sweet potatoes and plantains or bananas, if well tolerated. The added starch and fiber helps to feed the gut microflora, while the bone broth provides glycerin and healthy saturated fats.

Even on this diet, patients may not see any noticeable positive results for three months. Only if the fibromyalgia patient is getting remarkably worse during the first three months on the Paleo diet should he or she stop the protocol.

Once the fibromyalgia patient has been utilizing the strict Whole 30 Paleo diet for three months, the individual may begin re-adding foods to the diet.

Again, the process of restoring health is slow.

Since each person is a unique individual, and there is no "one size fits all" in the natural health community, customizing a specific Paleo diet protocol is paramount.

Paleo Recipes

Soup Recipes

Very Easy Extra Quick Tomato Soup

Serves 3

- 1 pack tomato passata
- equal amount of water
- 10 drops stevia
- basil leaves (optional)

Cut open pack of passata and put into a pan. Fill up the pack with water. Add to the pan. Add stevia and basil leaves.

Bring to the boil and then serve.

* This will freeze.

Tomato and Vegetable Soup

Serves 4

- 2 tablesp. olive oil
- 1 large onion chopped or 3-4 tablesp. frozen ready chopped onion
- 1 stick celery – chopped
- 1teasp. ready garlic puree
- 2 tins tomatoes
- 1 tablesp. tomato puree
- 300 ml chicken stock (use wheat/dairy free)
- 1 large carrot – chopped

1. Put oil in pan and gently fry the onion, carrot, celery and garlic for 5 minutes.
2. Add 2 tins tomatoes, tomato puree and chicken stock.
3. Simmer for 10 minutes, add salt and pepper to taste.
4. Whizz up in a blender till smooth. Reheat.

* This will freeze.

„Cream" Of Chicken Soup

Serves 3 – 4

- whole carcass of a roasted chicken
- 2 spring onions- finely sliced
- 200g cauliflower – cut into small florets
- 1 teasp. dried or 2 teasp. fresh herb of choice – e.g. coriander salt freshly ground black pepper

1. Remove any remaining meat from the carcass and keep to one side.
2. Put carcass in a pan with lid and just cover with water. Bring to boil and then simmer for 1 hour. (In a pressure cooker it would be 20 minutes). Strain stock through a sieve and discard the carcass.
3. Add spring onions, cauliflower and herbs into stock and simmer until cauliflower is soft – about 8-10 minutes.
4. Whizz up with a hand held blender, or put through a liquidizer, until smooth. Add water to get the consistency you want and add salt and pepper to taste. Add the chicken meat.
5. Reheat before serving.

* This will freeze.

Tomato and Basil Soup

Serves 6-8

- 1 onion – chopped
- 1 leek – sliced
- 1 courgette (zucchini) - chopped
- 1 large tin chopped tomatoes
- 1 small tin tomato puree
- 2 teasp. fresh basil chopped or 1 teasp. dried basil
- Salt and freshly ground black pepper
- 1/2 pint stock or water 5 drops stevia

1. Place all ingredients, except the stevia, in a large pan and bring to the boil. Simmer for 10-15 minutes till vegetables are soft.
2. Whizz up with a hand blender till smooth. Add more water if needed to get the consistency desired and add stevia. Adjust salt and pepper to taste.
3. Reheat before serving.

* This will freeze

Carrot and Coriander Soup

Serves 3-4

- 4 large carrots
- 1 large onion
- 2 pints chicken stock
- 1/2 stick celery
- 1 teasp. ready garlic paste
- Handful of fresh coriander
- Salt and freshly ground black pepper

1. Peel and slice carrots, celery and onions.
2. Put in large pan with the water, garlic, seasoning and stock. Bring to the boil and then reduce heat to simmer until vegetables are soft. Add the roughly chopped coriander.
3. Whizz up the mixture with a blender till smooth. Adjust seasoning and add some finely chopped coriander. Reheat.

* This will freeze.

* Adjust the amount of water to vegetables for a thicker or thinner soup according to your preference.

Super-Fast Tomato Soup

Serves 2-3

- 1 small tin tomato puree
- 5 tins of water (use the empty tomato paste tin)
- 1 stock cube (wheat and dairy free)
- 4 sweeteners or few drops of Stevia
- 2 tablesp. tomato ketchup

1. Place all ingredients in a pan and bring to the boil stirring occasionally.

* This will freeze

Spicy Carrot Soup

Serves 4

- 1 tablesp. oil
- 1 onion chopped or 3-4 tablesp. frozen chopped onion
- 1 level teasp. garlic puree
- 1 teasp. dried crushed chilies
- 1 teasp. curry powder
- 750. chopped carrots (frozen ready diced once are good)
- 1 crushed lemongrass stalk
- 1 tin coconut milk
- 500ml of stock

1. Heat oil in pan and gently cook the onion, garlic, chilies for 5 mins.
2. Stir in curry powder, carrots and lemongrass. Cover and cook on low heat for 10 mins. Add coconut milk and stock and simmer until carrots are soft.
3. Remove the lemongrass and whiz up till smooth. Reheat.

* This will freeze.

Italian Bean and Vegetable Soup

Serves 4

- 200g frozen mixed vegetables
- 410g tin borlotti beans – drained and rinsed
- 1 onion - chopped or 2 tablesp. frozen chopped onions
- 850ml hot vegetable stock – fresh, carton or from a stock cube (wheat and dairy free)
- 400g tin chopped tomatoes
- low fat cooking spray or 1 tablesp. oil

1. Heat a large, lidded saucepan and spritz with the cooking spray or add the oil.
2. Stir fry the onions over a high heat for 2-3 mins.
3. Add 4 tablesp. of the stock, cover the pan and gently cook onion till soft.
4. Mix in the tomatoes, vegetables, beans and remaining stock.
5. Put on the lid and simmer for 5 mins till vegetables are tender. Add salt and pepper to taste.

Serve with gram flour pancakes for a nutritious hearty meal.

* This will freeze.

Quick Pea Soup

Serves 3-4

- 1 small bag frozen peas
- Knorr chicken stock pot or any wheat free stock
- boiling water
- salt and freshly ground black pepper

1. Put peas in a saucepan and add the stock pot or enough stock to cover peas.
2. Just cover the peas with boiling water and simmer for a few minutes till peas are soft and cooked.
3. Use a hand blender to liquidize the peas completely.
4. Add salt and pepper to taste.
5. Add more boiling water if soup is too thick.

Lunch Recipes

Onion, Pepper, and Pea Tortilla

Serves 4

- 200g jar roasted red peppers, drained and sliced
- 300g frozen diced onion or 2 large onions chopped
- 2 teasp. garlic puree
- 5 eggs beaten
- 200g frozen peas

1. Spray a large non-stick frying pan with low-fat cooking spray. Add onion, peppers and peas and gently fry for 12 -15 mins until softened. Add garlic.
2. Preheat grill to medium hot.
3. Pour beaten eggs into pan and stir so that the vegetables are evenly spread though out the egg.
4. Cook gently till tortilla is set at the bottom.
5. Place pan under grill and cook till top is set and golden.

* Mushrooms can be added if liked.

Huevos Rancheros in a Hurry

Serves 4

- 2 red peppers
- 1 tablesp. olive oil
- 1 jar tomato and chili pasta sauce (wheat and dairy free)
- 4 eggs
- chopped fresh parsley or 1 teasp. dried parsley

1. Deseed and slice red peppers. Using a frying pan, fry in oil till softened.
2. Add tomato sauce and cook for 3-4 mins to thicken slightly.
3. Make 4 hollows in mixture and carefully crack an egg into each hollow.
4. Cover pan with a lid and cook on medium heat until eggs are cooked through.
5. Top with parsley and serve.

Healthy Veggie Sizzle

Serves 4

- 1 tablesp. olive oil
- 1 small onion chopped
- 3 courgette chopped
- 1 deseeded and chopped red pepper
- 2 tablesp. chopped basil leaves or 1 teasp. dried basil
- 4 eggs
- 150 g mushrooms chopped
- 1/2 green pepper
- 1/2 red pepper

1. Heat oil in frying pan. Fry all veggies till cooked and browned. Stir in basil.
2. Make 4 hollows in mixture and crack an egg into each.
3. Cover pan and cook on medium heat till eggs are cooked through.

Home-Made Sausage Patties

Serves 4

- 1 lb. wheat and dairy free pork sausage meat
- Pinch salt
- Ground black pepper (omit if liked)
- 1/2 onion finely chopped
- 1/2 teasp. any dried herb or 1 teasp. finely chopped fresh herbs (rosemary, parsley, basil, oregano etc.)

1. Mix all ingredients together in a bowl till well combined.
2. Damp your hands and then pull out a ball about the size of a golf ball. Roll till smooth, then flatten with the palm of your hand till about 1/2 inch thick.
3. Fry gently for about 4 -5 minutes on both sides till brown and the center is cooked through.

* These will freeze uncooked – lay on a cooling rack in freezer till frozen then put in freezer bag. Defrost in microwave before cooking. Good for breakfast, lunch or dinner.

Vegetable Omelet

For each person you will need:

- Heat oil in frying pan
- 1/4 large onion finely chopped
- Small amount of cabbage, finely sliced
- Few florets of broccoli chopped
- 1 tomato sliced
- 1 tablesp. oil
- 2 eggs
- Black pepper and salt

1. Lightly fry onion, cabbage, broccoli in a pan.
2. Then add tomato and fry for just a minute or so.
3. Then beat together eggs with black pepper and salt in a bowl with 2 tablesp. water, and pour over the veggies in the pan.
4. When it is cooked on one side, finish it off under a medium hot grill to cook the top half.

Serve hot with salad for lunch or main meal
Serve hot for breakfast.

Curried Eggs

Serves 2

- 1 egg
- 1 onion
- 1 tablesp. oil
- 1 fresh red chili or pinch of dried chili flakes
- 2 teasp. turmeric
- 2 teasp. cumin
- 400g tin chopped tomatoes
- 100g frozen or fresh spinach
- 100g kefir

1. Put eggs in a pan and cover with water.
2. Bring to the boil, then reduce to a simmer for 8 minutes to hard boil them.
3. Pour off hot water and fill pan with cold water.
4. In a separate pan, add the oil and spices, and dice or slice the onion according to preference. Cook on a medium heat for a few minutes to soften the onions.
5. Pour the chopped tomatoes over the now-spicy onions, and add the frozen spinach. Bring to the boil, then reduce the heat and leave to simmer.
6. Peel and halve the eggs and add to the sauce with the kefir, stir in.
7. Heat through, and serve on a bed of mashed cooked cauliflower.

Egg "Pancakes"

- 2 eggs per person
- Your choice of frying oil (olive, coconut, dairy-free spread, etc.)
- Toppings of your choice (e.g. fried peppers, wheat free chipolatas, bacon, allowed fruit, kefir, nuts, high cocoa chocolate chips, coconut cream)

1. Break the eggs into a mug and whisk with a fork.
2. Heat a frying pan with a little of your choice of frying oil.
3. Tip the eggs into the pan and swirl until the pan is coated.
4. Cook gently over a low heat until the eggs are cooked.
5. Serve hot with the toppings of your choice.

This makes for an extremely easy and stone age friendly pancake substitute!

Very versatile and works well with sweet or savory toppings.

Bean Fry

Serves 2-3

- 1 onion
- 1 green, orange or red pepper few mushrooms
- 1 tin red kidney beans
- 1-2 tablesp. oil, lard or dripping mixed herbs

1. Chop vegetables.
2. Fry in oil, lard or dripping till softened and golden brown.
3. Add large pinch herbs and drained beans. Heat through.

Hummus

- 14 0z/400g tin chick peas
- 2-3 tablesp. tahini
- 1/2-1 teasp. salt
- 1 tablesp. olive oil
- Approx. 3 tablesp. chickpea water (from tin)
- Juice of one lemon or 3-4 tablesp. bottled lemon juice
- 1-3 peeled, sliced cloves of garlic or 3 teasp. ready garlic in a tube
Black pepper
- Paprika

1. Drain chickpeas, reserving liquid.
2. In a food processor, blend chickpeas, lemon juice, garlic, salt, pepper, tahini and oil and blend to a thick paste.
3. Add enough chick pea water to make the consistency smooth (it should still be firm enough to use as a spread).
4. Serve sprinkled with paprika.

This is good on buckwheat crispbreads, bread substitutes or oatcakes. This will freeze or keep in the fridge in an air tight container for up to a week

* This will freeze.

Devilled Eggs

Serves 3 for a lunch dish but more for a snack

- 6 eggs – hard boiled, peeled and halved lengthways.

Pesto
- a handful of fresh basil, chopped
- 2-3 tablesp. extra virgin olive oil
- sea salt – to taste
- 1 tablesp. pine nuts.

1. Make the pesto by combining all ingredients, except the eggs, and mixing well.
2. Remove the hard egg yolk and put in a bowl with 3 tablesp. of the pesto. Mix well together.
3. Heap the egg yolk and pesto mix in the holes left by the egg yolk.
4. Serve cold as an appetizer, canapé, snack or a lunch dish.

Pesto can be kept in the fridge for at least a week. So you could make twice the recipe and use as a salad dressing.

The filled eggs could be kept overnight in the fridge if covered with cling film.

Meat Recipes

Beef Stew

Serves 4

- 450g lean rump/ silverside or topside beef
- 200g onions chopped
- 1 400g tin chopped tomatoes
- 1 green or red pepper chopped
- 1 leek sliced
- Other vegetables such as celery or courgette
- 20mls vegetable oil, lard or dripping
- 2 cloves garlic or 1 tablesp. ready chopped garlic
- 1 bay leaf
- 1 teasp. dried Italian herbs or oregano.
- 200g carrots sliced
- 150g mushrooms sliced

1. Gently fry garlic in oil, lard or dripping for 1 minute. Add onions, mushrooms and fry for 1 minute. Then add meat and fry for another minute till browned.
2. Add tomatoes, carrots and cook for two hours on a low heat with the pan covered, or for 1 hour if pressure cooked.
3. Add all other ingredients and cook for a further hour in a covered pan or another 15 minutes in the pressure cooker.

Serve with green vegetables.

* This will freeze.

Banger Surprise

Serves 4

- 8 wheat-free sausages – Black Farmer or CO-OP own, debbie and andrews. (debbie and andrews are suitable for those with Fermenting Gut)
- 1 red pepper – deseeded and chopped into large pieces
- 1 green pepper- deseeded and chopped into large pieces
- 2 red onions – chopped roughly
- 4-5 cloves of garlic – peeled but leave whole
- 2 tablesp. olive oil, lard or dripping

1. Light oven gas 5, 375F, 190C.
2. Use an open oven proof dish and add all ingredients.
3. Drizzle with the olive oil, lard or dripping
4. Bake for 45 minutes till sausages are brown and cooked through and the vegetables are soft.

Serve with any leafy greens or a green salad.

* This will freeze.

Beef Burgers

Serves 4

- 500g or 1 lb. lean minced beef
- 1 onion finely chopped
- 1 level teasp. mixed herbs
- 1 clove garlic crushed or 1 teasp. ready garlic from tube – (opt)
- Salt and pepper

1. Mix all ingredients together well.
2. Shape into burgers using damp hands or a burger maker – makes 8.
3. Fry slowly in a frying pan or on a BBQ till browned and cooked through.
4. Serve with a large mixed salad drizzled with olive oil.

These can be eaten for breakfast too.

Burgers can be frozen raw on a cooling rack and then stored in freezer bags. Cook from frozen.

Beef Burgers 2

Serves 4-6

- 500g minced beef
- 1/2 tablesp. rosemary (finely chopped)
- 1/2 tablesp. thyme (finely chopped)
- 1/2 tablesp. sage (finely chopped)
- 2 cloves of garlic (minced)
- 1/2 teasp. salt
- large pinch baking powder
- 1 tablesp. solid cooking fat like lard or dripping

1. Combine all the ingredients (except fat) in a bowl.
2. Divide into 6 patties.
3. Heat the oil in a frying pan over a medium heat and cook for approx. 5 mins. per side.

These will freeze raw on a cooling rack. Burgers can either be thawed or cooked from frozen.

Beef Curry Stir Fry

Serves 4

- 1 tablesp. oil, lard or dripping – choose one you like
- 1 tablesp. red or yellow Thai curry paste
- 400g lean minced beef
- 2 tablesp. Thai fish sauce
- Few drops Stevia
- 4 baby pak choi, quartered
- 4 spring onions
- 1/2 white cabbage or small cauliflower

1. Heat the oil, lard or dripping in a large wok or frying pan. Fry the curry paste for 1 minute. Add the beef and fry for 3 minutes.
2. Add 100ml water, the fish sauce and Stevia to the pan and simmer for 5 minutes. Add the pak choi and spring onions and cook for another minute or until wilted.
3. Serve over a bed of steamed or boiled white cabbage or a bed of mashed cauliflower.

* The meat curry will freeze, but not the cabbage or cauliflower.

Beef Goulash

Serves 6

- 1kg / 2.2 lbs. good braising steak, preferably chuck steak
- 1 tablesp. oil, lard or dripping
- 3 medium onions, cut into 12 wedges
- 3 garlic cloves or 3 teasp. ready garlic from tube
- 2 teasp. hot smoked paprika
- 1 tablesp. paprika
- 600ml beef stock (wheat and dairy free)
- 400g tin chopped tomatoes
- 2 tablesp. tomato puree
- 2 bay leaves
- 1 red pepper
- 1 green pepper
- 1 orange/yellow pepper
- salt and freshly ground black pepper

1. Light oven 170C, 375F, gas 3 1/2.
2. Chop the beef into 1 inch chunks. Season well with salt and pepper.
3. Heat the oil, lard or dripping in a large flame proof casserole dish or a large wok or frying pan. Fry beef over high heat till nicely browned.
4. Add the onions and cook with the beef for 5 minutes until softened. Add the garlic and fry for another minute.
5. Sprinkle both paprikas over the meat. Add stock, tomatoes, tomato puree and bay leaves. Cover casserole with lid or transfer beef mix to an oven proof casserole and cook for 1 1/2 hours.
6. Remove core and seeds from the peppers and cut into 1-inch chunks.
7. After beef has cooked for 1 1/2 hours, add the peppers and put back in the oven for another hour or until the meat is very tender.

* This will freeze.

Braised Silverside (Beef)

Serves 6-8

- 3 medium onions – peeled and sliced
- 1 large tin chopped tomatoes
- 3-3 1/2 lbs. silverside (joint of beef)
- 1 level teasp. mixed dried herbs
- 250g French beans or green beans
- Salt and pepper

1. Light oven 300F, gas mark 2, 160C or get out slow cooker.
2. Place sliced onions in the bottom of the slow cooker crock or an oven proof casserole with lid big enough to take the joint.
3. Add chopped tomatoes. Place meat on top of vegetables and sprinkle with mixed herbs and salt and pepper.
4. Cover and cook in oven for 3 1/4 - 3 3/4 hours or 12 hours in slow cooker.
5. Trim ends of French beans and add to casserole. Baste meat with juices from the vegetables and cover and cook for a further 3/4 hour in oven or a couple of hours in the slow cooker until the meat is tender and the beans are cooked.
6. Remove meat and carve into slices. Serve with other allowed vegetables and the tomato and onions as a sauce.

* This will freeze.

Pot Roast Brisket

Serves 4-6

This is delicious served with green vegetables for a different Sunday Roast.

- A large piece of rolled, boned brisket. (Brisket is a cheap cut of beef which has a delicious flavor, but needs long slow cooking)
- 2 onions or 1/2 packet ready prepared diced frozen onions
- 1 leek (opt)
- 2 sticks celery (opt)
- 2 teasp. garlic puree (opt)
- 2 beef stock cubes – wheat free 3/4 pint boiling water
- 1 level teasp. mixed herbs
- 2 dried bay leaves
- 2 large carrots
- Selection of root vegetables or a packet of ready prepared root vegetables or for fermenting gut diet add other allowed vegetables like courgette, aubergine etc. instead of the root vegetables

1. Peel, chop all vegetables into small pieces and put into a slow cooker or an oven proof dish.
2. Make up the stock cubes with boiling water and add garlic puree. Add to pot.
3. Place brisket on top of vegetables and put on lid.
4. If cooking in an oven, gas mark 4, 350F, 180C place on top shelf and cook for 4- 5 hours.
5. Slice meat and serve vegetables and gravy in the pot it was cooked in.
6. If cooking in a slow cooker, then allow 12- 16 hours. It can be put on the night before and left.

If you like thicker gravy, remove meat onto a plate, then mix 2 level tablesp. gram flour with some cold water and then add the hot gravy to the cold mix. Stir well and put in a pan and bring to the boil, stirring all the time till it thickens. Pour gravy back into the pot of vegetables and stir in.

Left over vegetables and gravy can be whizzed up in a liquidizer (remove bay leaves first) and more water added to make a tasty soup. Add plenty of salt and pepper to taste.

Lamb and Herb Burgers

Serves 4

- 450 g lean lamb mince
- 1 clove garlic or 1 heaped teasp. garlic puree
- 2 level teasp. dried rosemary
- 1 medium finely chopped onion
- salt and pepper

1. Mix all ingredients together.
2. With damp hands, shape mixture into 4 burgers.
3. Chill for 20 minutes.
4. Grill for 6-8 minutes on each side till juices run clear. Or cook on BBQ.

These are good served in gram flour pancakes (Stone Age only) with salad.

These will freeze cooked and easily reheated in the microwave or frozen raw and either defrosted before cooking or cook from frozen.

Meat and Egg Loaf

Serves 4

- 350 g lean minced beef
- 1 level tablesp. tomato puree
- salt and pepper
- pinch grated nutmeg
- pinch dried thyme
- 1 large egg, fresh
- 2 hard boiled eggs
- 1 small onion, finely chopped
- pinch all spice
- 1 level teasp. finely chopped parsley or half teasp. dried parsley
- 1 tablesp. Worcestershire sauce

1. Light oven 190C, 375F, gas 5.
2. Mix all ingredients, except the hard boiled eggs, in a large bowl.
3. Shape into a flat rectangle, and place hard eggs down the center.
4. Roll up meat into a roll and place in a greased loaf tin. Bake for 1 hour.

Serve hot with vegetables or cold with salad.

* This will freeze.

Stuffed Peppers

Serves 3

Sauce
- 1 onion chopped
- 400g tin of tomatoes
- few drops Stevia
- 1/2 teasp. Italian seasoning
- 150 ml boiling water.
- 4 mushrooms chopped

Peppers
- 3 green peppers
- 1 medium onion
- salt and pepper
- 225g lean minced beef
- 1 small egg, beaten

Light oven 160C, 325F, Gas 3

Sauce
1. Fry onions and mushrooms in a teasp. oil till soft.
2. Add tomatoes, stock pot, water and salt and pepper.
3. Simmer over a low heat for 15 mins.

Peppers
1. Cut peppers in half lengthways and de-seed. Place in a pan of boiling water and simmer for 5 minutes. Drain well.
2. Grate the onion and mix with the beef, egg and salt and pepper. Fill the peppers with this mixture.
3. Place in an ovenproof dish and pour over the sauce.
4. Cover and bake for 1 hour.

Serve with vegetables or salad.

Kebabs

Serves 4

- 500g or 1 lb. pork loin cut into cubes
- Selection of vegetables cut into chunks – onions, courgette, tomatoes, green, red, yellow peppers, cloves of garlic, mushrooms, etc.
- Cajun rub (if liked)
- Metal or wooden skewers pre-soaked in water

1. Prepare pork and vegetables.
2. Coat pork cubes with dry rub and a few drops of Stevia.
3. Fill skewers with vegetables and meat.
4. Brush with olive oil, lard or dripping and grill on BBQ till browned and the meat is cooked through.

Serve with mixed salad drizzled with olive oil.

Pork, Herb and Apple Burgers

Serves 4

- 450 g lean pork mince
- 1 clove garlic or 1 heaped teasp. garlic puree
- 2 level teasp. dried rosemary
- 1 medium finely chopped onion
- Salt and pepper
- 1 peeled, grated medium cooking apple or 1 large eating apple or 3 tablesp. dried apple cubes

1. Mix all ingredients together.
2. With damp hands, shape mixture into 4 burgers.
3. Chill for 20 minutes.
4. Grill for 6-8 minutes on each side till juices run clear. Or cook on BBQ.

* These will freeze either raw or cooked.

Meat Loaf

Serves 4

- 450g lean finely minced beef salt and pepper
- pinch of mixed herbs
- 1 egg white
- 1 medium tomato, finely chopped
- 1 medium onion, finely chopped
- 1 small carrot, grated

1. Light oven 190C, 375F, Gas 5.
2. Grease and line a loaf tin with greaseproof paper or parchment.
3. Put all ingredients into a mixing bowl and mix well.
4. Put mixture into the loaf tin.
5. Bake for 1 hour.
6. Serve hot with vegetables or cold with salad.

* This will freeze.

Home-made Sausage Patties

Serves 4

- 1 lb. wheat and dairy free pork sausage meat
- Pinch salt
- Ground black pepper (omit if liked)
- 1/2 onion finely-chopped
- 1/2 teasp. any dried herb or 1 teasp. finely chopped fresh herbs (rosemary, parsley, basil, oregano, etc.)

1. Mix all ingredients together in a bowl till well combined.
2. Damp your hands and then pull out a ball about the size of a golf ball. Roll till smooth, then flatten with the palm of your hand till about 1/2 inch thick.
3. Fry gently for about 4 -5 minutes on both sides till brown and the center is cooked through.

These will freeze uncooked – lay on a cooling rack in freezer till frozen then put in freezer bag. Defrost in microwave before cooking. Good for breakfast, lunch or dinner.

Tex Mex Chili with Chili Cream

Serves 4

- 3 large red chilies
- 1 tablesp. olive oil, lard or dripping
- 1 large onion roughly chopped
- 2 large garlic cloves or 2 teasp. ready garlic from tube
- 1 red pepper, deseeded and cut into chunks
- 1 orange pepper, deseeded and cut into chunks
- 2 tablesp. ground cumin
- 1 teasp. ground cinnamon
- 1 tablesp. paprika
- 500g minced beef or Quorn mince
- 200g tin chopped tomatoes with chili and garlic
- 500g passata with herbs
- 400g tin kidney beans
- 6 tablesp. soy yoghurt or Kefir

1. Deseed and finely chop 2 of the chilies.
2. Put the oil, lard or dripping in a pan and fry the chilies, onion, garlic and peppers for 5 minutes until softened.
3. Add the cumin, cinnamon, and paprika and cook for 1-2 minutes, stirring well.
4. Stir in the mince or Quorn, tomatoes, passata and beans and 300ml of cold water. Bring to the boil and simmer for 20 minutes.
5. Use long handled tongs to cook the remaining chili directly over an open flame, turning until charred.
6. Place in a plastic food bag and seal and leave to steam for 10 minutes. Remove the blackened skin and seeds, mash the flesh and stir into the yoghurt or Kefir.

Serve meat over a bed of cooked shredded white cabbage or cooked mashed cauliflower and pour over some of the chili cream.
This is very spicy. Use fewer chilies if you don't want it too hot.

Lamb and Vegetable Curry

Serves 4

- 2 tablesp. oil, lard or dripping
- 2 onions, peeled and chopped
- 400g diced lamb
- 5 cm. root ginger, peeled and grated
- 4 tablesp. Rogan josh paste
- 400g tin tomatoes
- 600ml chicken stock made from Knorr stock cube or 600 ml chicken stock made from a chicken carcass for fermenting gut
- 125g yellow split peas
- 200g carrots, sliced thinly
- 250g green beans, halved
- 5 tablesp. Kefir or soy yoghurt
- 8 radishes chopped (opt)

1. Light oven 180C, gas mark 4.
2. Heat oil, lard or dripping in a large flame proof casserole or in a large pan and fry onions for 5 minutes to soften.
3. Add the lamb and cook for 10 minutes to lightly brown.
4. Stir in the ginger, curry paste and cook for a couple of minutes. Add tomatoes and chicken stock.
5. Add salt and pepper to taste and the yellow split peas, green beans and carrots. Bring to the boil.
6. Put the flame proof casserole in the oven or transfer the contents of the pan into an oven-proof dish. Cover with a lid and cook for 50 – 60 minutes in the oven until the meat and vegetables are tender.
7. Serve with a generous dollop of kefir or soy yoghur* and sprinkled with radishes.

This would be good on either a bed of finely chopped cooked white cabbage or mashed cooked cauliflower.

Lamb Meat Balls/Burgers

Serves 4

Meatball/burger ingredients:
- 500g ground lamb
- 2 tablesp. Kalamata olives (finely chopped)
- 2 cloves garlic (crushed)
- Zest of 1/2 lemon
- 1/2 teaspoon cinnamon
- 1/2 teaspoon sea salt
- 1/2 tablesp. avocado oil / hard cooking fat like lard or dripping

Optional meatball juice:
- 200ml bone broth 1/2 lemon, juiced

1. Mix all the ball/burger ingredients together and form into 1-inch balls (or burgers).
2. Heat oil / fat in large frying pan over a medium high heat and fry meatballs for a couple of minutes on each „side" until all well browned (around 10 mins in total). If making burgers fry on both sides for 4-5 mins depending on thickness.
3. If using the jus set aside the balls on a warm plate, turn the heat to low and add the jus ingredients. It will boil very vigorously due to the hot pan, so be careful. Deglaze pan, leave for a minute or two and then spoon over balls.

* The meatballs will freeze either cooked or raw.

Chili Con Carne

Serves 4

- 1 tablesp. oil, lard or dripping
- 2 large onions chopped
- 2 cloves garlic crushed or 2 teasp. ready garlic from tube
- 500g or 1 lb. minced beef
- 2 teasp. chili powder
- 1 teasp. cumin powder (opt)
- 1 x 65 g tomato puree
- 1 x 425g tin red kidney beans, drained
- 300ml (1/2 pint) beef stock (use 1/2 Knorr Stock pot and 1/2 pint water)
- 100g (4 oz.) mushrooms
- Salt and pepper

1. Dry fry the minced beef in a large pan till browned. Add the garlic and onions and fry for a further 2 minutes.
2. Add all other ingredients (except kidney beans) and bring to the boil.
3. Simmer for 1/2 - 3/4 hour with a lid. Stir every now and then.
4. Add kidney beans and bring to boil to warm beans through.

Serve on a bed of cooked shredded white cabbage or a bed of cooked mashed cauliflower with green vegetables and /or a mixed salad.

* This freezes.

Moroccan Meatballs

Serves 4

Meatballs:
- 500g minced beef
- 3 tablesp. oatmeal
- 1 egg
- Salt and pepper
- 1tablesp. chopped parsley or 1 level teasp. dried parsley

1. Mix all together and shape into balls with damp hands. Cook as required.

* These will freeze raw or cooked.

Sauce
- 100g dried ready to eat apricots
- halved 25 flaked almonds
- 1 tbsp. olive oil, lard or dripping
- 1 onion chopped
- 400g tin chopped tomatoes with garlic handful fresh or 2 teasp. dried coriander
- 1 level teasp. cinnamon

1. Fry meatballs in the oil, lard or dripping for 10 mins. turning until cooked. Remove from pan.
2. Add onion and cook until soft.
3. Add apricots, cinnamon and tomatoes.
4. Half fill the can with water and add to pan.
5. Bring to the boil, then simmer for 5 mins.
6. Return meatballs to the pan and heat through.
7. Sprinkle over the almonds and coriander and serve with other allowed vegetables.

* This will freeze.

Sausage and Bean Pot

Serves 4

- 4 large sausages – wheat and dairy free
- 200g frozen diced onion or two large onions, peeled and chopped
227g (jar) sundried tomato paste
- 1 dried bay leaf (opt)
- 1 can haricot beans drained
- 1/2 teasp. dried thyme
- 1 teasp. dried rosemary
- 400ml water

1. Fry sausages in non- stick frying pan till golden brown and cooked. Remove sausages from pan and discard most of the fat.
2. Cook onion until soft but not browned.
3. Add tomato paste and cook for two mins.
4. Add the beans, water, herbs, season well with salt and pepper. Simmer for 10 mins.
5. Slice sausages and add to pan. Simmer until the sauce is thick enough to coat the back of a spoon.
6. Serve with a green vegetable.

* This will freeze.

Simple Pork Stir – Fry

Serves 4

- 1 tablesp. gram flour
- salt and black pepper
- 600g pork tenderloin thinly sliced
- 2 tablesp. oil, lard or dripping
- 3 carrots cut into thin batons
- 1 red and 1 green pepper thinly sliced
- 24 French beans
- 20 baby button mushrooms sliced
- Juice of 1 lemon or 3-4 tablesp. bottled
- 1 tablesp. dairy/wheat free soy sauce
- 3 teasp. fish sauce (opt)

1. Put the flour into a re-sealable food bag, add salt and pepper. Shake well. Add the pork and shake well to coat the pork. Put into a sieve to remove any excess flour.
2. Pour the oil, lard or dripping into a large frying pan or wok and heat to a high heat. Add the pork and fry for 1-2 mins until brown.
3. Add the veg. and toss. Add lemon juice, fish and soy sauces and fry for 5-10 mins. till veg. is cooked but still slightly crisp and the pork is cooked through.

Can be served on a bed of cooked shredded white cabbage, or cooked mashed cauliflower.
This is very tasty and quick to do. Sliced chicken could be used instead of pork.

Sausage, Lamb and Pineapple Casserole

Serves 4

- 4 small lamb chops
- 4 wheat free sausages
- 50g mushrooms
- 350ml stock (made from wheat and dairy free cube)
- 4 pineapple rings

1. Light oven gas 4, 350F, 180C.
2. Grill sausages and cut into three.
3. Place lamb chops in flat casserole dish. Place a ring of pineapple on top of each chop with a whole mushroom in the hole in the ring.
4. Chop rest of mushrooms and arrange round the chops with the sausage pieces.
5. Pour in stock and bake in oven for 1 hour 15 minutes.

Serve with green vegetables.

Thai Beef Salad

Serves 4

- 2.5cm piece of root ginger, finely grated or 4 teasp. ready chopped ginger from jar
- 1 stick of lemon grass, finely sliced (outer leaves removed)
- 1 tablesp. fish sauce
- 1 tablesp. wheat free soy sauce
- 2 teasp. sesame oil
- juice of 1 lime
- 1 red chili, deseeded and finely chopped
- 2 x 240 g rump steaks, trimmed of fat
- 10cm piece cucumber cut into batons
- 100g salad leaves
- 80g cherry tomatoes
- 80g bean sprouts
- Handful each of fresh coriander, basil, and mint leaves roughly torn

1. Mix the ginger, lemon grass, fish sauce, soy sauce, oil, lime juice and chili together. Pour half the marinade over the steaks and marinade overnight or from the morning till the evening.
2. Preheat the grill to high. Remove the steak from the marinade (discard this marinade) and grill on each side for 2-4 minutes according to taste. Set aside for 10 minutes before slicing.
3. Place the other half of the marinade in a bowl and add the steak and the rest of the ingredients.
4. Toss to coat before serving.

This could be expensive because of the cost of good beef.

Easy Cassoulet

Serves 4

- 2 tablesp. olive oil, lard or dripping
- 4 wheat and dairy free sausages
- 4 boneless, skinless chicken thighs opened out flat
- 1 large onion peeled and chopped
- 2 celery sticks washed and chopped
- 2 teasp. paprika
- 2 x 400g tins chopped tomatoes with garlic and herbs
- 2 x 400g tins cannellini beans, rinsed and drained

1. Heat the oil, lard or dripping in a large saucepan. Add the sausages and the chicken thighs and fry for 5 minutes until browned. Remove from the pan and slice the sausages.
2. Add the onion and celery to the pan and fry 2-3 minutes till slightly softened. Add the paprika and return the sausages and chicken to the pan.
3. Add the tomatoes, beans, salt and pepper. Bring to the boil and reduce heat to simmer for 20 minutes.

This would be good served with green vegetables on a bed of either mashed cauliflower or white cabbage.
Bread substitutes could be eaten with this too.

Succulent Pork Chops

Serves 4

- 4 pork chops
- 4 tablesp. rolled oats (whizzed up in a grinder to a flour) or gram flour 1-2 teasp. dried herbs and spices – choose any of your favorites
- Salt and freshly ground black pepper

1. Light oven 200C, 400F, gas mark 6.
2. Mix oats or gram flour with herbs and spices, salt and pepper. Put on a large plate.
3. Dip pork chops in the mixture to coat each side - make sure the meat is all covered.
4. Place coated chops in a greased oven proof dish and bake for 30 minutes until meat is tender and cooked through.

This is also good on a bed of roasted vegetables.

Chicken Recipes

Thai Red Curry

Serves 2-3

- 1 onion or two tablesp. ready chopped frozen onion
- 1 teasp. ready garlic
- 3 tablesp. red curry paste
- 1 tablesp. groundnut or olive oil
- 400g tin chopped tomatoes
- 2 x 400ml coconut milk
- 250ml fish or chicken stock (for wheat free check label)
- 150 g sugar snap peas
- 4 tablesp. fish sauce
- salt and black pepper
- 400 g raw prawns or chicken diced
- 12 button mushrooms halved
- juice of 1 lime or 2 tablesp. lime juice
- 400g butternut squash peeled and diced into 1/4-inch cubes

Instead of mushrooms and butternut squash for those with fermenting gut, substitute courgette.

1. Whiz up the onion, garlic and curry paste in a blender or finely chop onion and mix with garlic and curry paste.
2. Pour oil in saucepan and when hot add the paste and tomatoes. Cook for 5 mins. stirring all the time.
3. Add the coconut milk and the squash. Bring to the boil and simmer for 10-15 mins till squash is tender.
4. Add sugar snap peas and fish sauce. Add salt and pepper.
5. Add prawns or chicken to curry sauce and cook till tender – prawns are ready when they go pink – do not overcook as they go hard.

Can be served on a bed of cooked mashed cauliflower.

Chicken Kievs

For each person you need:
- 1 chicken breast
- 1 teasp. dairy-free margarine
- small amount garlic puree
- pinch dried herbs – Italian herbs or any you like
- 1 slice bacon

1. Light oven gas mark 5, 175C, 375 F.
2. Grease a baking sheet.
3. Mix margarine, garlic and herbs to form a paste.
4. Cut sideways into the chicken breast to make a pocket and fill with paste.
5. Wrap a slice of bacon round the breast to seal the pocket.
6. Bake for 30-35 minutes until cooked through.

This very tasty and so easy to prepare. Would be nice with vegetables or salad.

Spicy Chicken with Vegetable Sauce

Serves 4

For the spicy chicken:
- 4 chicken breasts or thighs
- 2 garlic cloves crushed or two teasp. ready garlic from tube
- 1 lemon, juice only or three tablesp. ready lemon juice out of a bottle
- 1 heaped teasp. paprika
- 1 teasp. ground cumin
- pinch cayenne pepper
- 1 teasp. turmeric
- Sea salt and freshly ground black pepper
- 1tbs olive oil

For the sauce:
- 2 tbsp. olive oil
- 1 garlic clove crushed or 1 teasp. ready garlic from tube
- 1 aubergine chopped
- 1 red onion chopped
- 2 courgette chopped
- 1 red pepper deseeded and chopped
- 1 x 400g/14oz tin tomatoes
- sprig fresh oregano
- small handful chopped flat leaf parsley
- 1 lemon, grated zest only

For the spicy chicken:

1. Mix all the ingredients except the oil together in a mixing bowl and mix to ensure the chicken is completely coated in the ingredients.
2. Marinade for at least 3 hours or overnight.
3. To cook the chicken, heat a griddle pan, remove the chicken from the marinade and rub all over with the olive oil.
4. Place on the griddle and cook for about 15minutes for breast and 20minutes for thighs, turning once or twice. Ensure juices run clear.

For the vegetable sauce:

1. Heat the olive oil in a wide pan and fry the garlic for 1 minute until soft.
2. Add the aubergine, onions, courgette and red pepper to the pan and fry for 20 minutes until softened, stirring regularly.
3. Stir in the tomatoes and oregano and cook for a further 20 minutes until reduced and thick.
4. Mix together the parsley and lemon zest in a small bowl and stir this through the vegetables and serve with the chicken.

This would be good served on a bed of finely shredded and cooked white cabbage or mashed cooked cauliflower.

The vegetable sauce would be good with pork chops, wheat free sausages or plain chicken.

* This would freeze.

Ham, Chicken & Tarragon Pie

Serves 4-6

Filling:
- 1.5 kg Ham Hock
- 6 Whole Chicken Legs
- 2 Carrots
- 2 Stick Celery
- 1 Onion (halved)
- 1 Bouquet Garni (bag of herbs)
- Filtered Water

Sauce:
- 1 tablesp. Fresh Tarragon (chopped)
- 1-2 tablesp. Arrowroot (mixed with a splash of cold water)

Topping:
- 2 Cauliflowers (florets removed)
- 2 tablesp. Olive Oil, or Ghee
- Sea Salt

1. Remove the meats from the fridge and bring to room temperature (30 minutes).
2. Place ham in a saucepan, cover with water and bring to the boil. Pour off the water and rinse the ham.
3. Place all the filling ingredients into a slow cooker, or large casserole. Add enough water to just cover them all.
4. In the slow cooker, crock pot, cook on high for 2 - 3 hours, or simmer in casserole for 1 – 2 hours until the meats are cooked (you may have to remove the chicken legs earlier).
5. For the topping, boil the cauliflower florets in plenty of salted water for around 10 minutes until tender. Drain thoroughly and remove as much water as possible from them with kitchen towel. Return to the saucepan and mash with the oil/ghee and season to taste. Set aside.

6. Once cooked remove the meat and set aside to cool a little. Throw away the vegetables/herbs and pour the broth into a degreasing jug. Pour 500ml into a saucepan (the remaining broth can be frozen for future use) and place over a medium/high heat to boil for 20 minutes or so, to reduce the liquid by half.
7. Meanwhile remove the fat/skin from the meat and throw away. Strip the meat from the bones, arrange in a large pie dish and sprinkle with the tarragon.
8. Once reduced, turn the heat down to a simmer under the broth and whisk in enough arrowroot mixture to form a thick gravy. Check for seasoning (should be salty enough from the ham).
9. Pour the gravy over the meat and top with the mash.
10. At this point the pie can be refrigerated, or frozen. The pie should be at room temperature before the next stage of cooking.
11. Place the pie in a preheated oven for around 20 minutes at 180C. And then under the grill for 5 minutes to brown.

Serve with greens of your choice.

* This will freeze.

Chicken Curry

Serves 4

- 4 small skinned chicken breasts (halved) or 8 skinned thighs
- 1 onion (peeled)
- 3 large garlic cloves (peeled)
- 5 cm cube ginger (peeled & roughly chopped)
- 2 tablesp. coconut oil
- 1 tablesp. turmeric
- 1 tablesp. coconut flour
- 100g creamed coconut (from a block) or 1 tin coconut cream
- 100-120ml chicken stock
- 1 teasp. salt
- 1/2 teasp. ground black pepper
- 2 tablesp. fresh lime/lemon juice
- Chopped fresh coriander
- 2 green chilies (deseeded & finely chopped)
- 1 tablesp. ground cumin
- 2 teasp. ground coriander
- 1/2 teasp. turmeric
- 1/2 teasp. cayenne
- 1/2 teasp. paprika
- 1 tablesp. tomato puree

1. Add the onion, garlic and ginger to a food processor and whizz until all very finely chopped.
2. Heat oil in a frying pan over a low-medium heat and add the onion mixture. Allow to cook for around 10 minutes stirring occasionally.
3. Reduce the heat to low and add the coconut flour and turmeric. Add a little water to loosen the paste and cook for a couple of minutes.
4. Mix the creamed coconut with enough hot water to make a thick cream. Add the coconut cream, stock, salt and pepper to the pan and bring to the simmer.
5. Add chicken pieces to a slow cooker/casserole (with lid) and cover with the sauce.

6. Slow cooker; cook on low for 5-6 hours, or high for 2-3 hours. Casserole; cover with a circle of greaseproof paper sitting on top of the mixture and then the lid, cook for 1.5 hours at 150C, gas 4.
7. Once cooked stir in the lime juice and serve with veg of your choice and the fresh coriander sprinkled on top.

Oriental Chicken

Serves 2

- 1 large tin bean sprouts or fresh bean sprouts
- 1 large onion, chopped
- 225 cooked chicken
- salt and pepper
- 3 tablesp. wheat free soy sauce
- 120 g mushrooms, sliced

1. Fry the onions in the soy sauce till tender.
2. Add the mushrooms and cook gently for a further 2-3 minutes.
3. Add the bean sprouts and chicken, heat thoroughly stirring all the time.

Serve with vegetables or salad.

Moroccan Chicken

Serves 4

- 1 Jar Tagine Sauce
- 4 chicken breasts
- 1 1/2 green, red peppers chopped finely (or equivalent ready frozen peppers)
- 100g streaky bacon – chopped finely
- 1 onion or 3-4 tablesp. ready chopped frozen onion
- 100 g roughly chopped ready to eat or dried apricots
- olive oil, lard or dripping
- dried garlic powder or 1 teasp. ready tube garlic

1. Light oven gas reg 5, 190C or 375F.
2. Fry chicken breasts in a little olive oil, lard or dripping with garlic to brown the meat. Put into a flat oven proof dish.
3. Fry onions, peppers, bacon, apricots and garlic in pan with a little olive oil, lard or dripping. Add sauce and 1 sauce jar of water and heat through. Pour over chicken.
4. Bake for 25-30 mins till chicken is cooked through.

Can be served on a bed of cooked shredded white cabbage, or cooked mashed cauliflower.

* This will freeze.

Hawaiian Chicken

Serves 4

- 4 chicken breasts or 8 thighs
- 2 tablesp. gram
- 1 teasp. paprika pepper
- large pinch salt
- large pinch black pepper
- 2-3 tablesp. oil, lard or dripping
- 1 teasp. grated orange rind
- 125ml orange juice
- large tin crushed pineapple
- 1 large orange sliced

1. Light oven gas 4, 180C, 350F. Grease a flat oven proof casserole dish.
2. Mix flour, paprika, salt and pepper in a bag and toss chicken to coat.
3. Fry chicken in the oil, lard or dripping in a frying pan till browned. Arrange in bottom of dish.
4. Sprinkle with orange rind, orange juice and crushed pineapple.
5. Bake for 45mins – 1 hour. 5 minutes before end of cooking time arrange orange slices over the top and reheat till piping hot.

Serve with green vegetables or crispy green salad.
This is very tasty and easy and quick to make.

Zesty Chicken Stir Fry

Serves 2

- 1 tablesp. soy sauce
- Juice of 1 small orange or 2 tablesp. orange juice from carton
- 2 tablesp. oil, lard or dripping
- 1 large chicken breast cut into chunks
- 1 onion chopped or 4 tablesp. frozen chopped onion
- 150g mange tout
- 1 red pepper chopped
- Any other vegetables like bean sprouts, bamboo shoots and/or water chestnuts (these can be bought in tins separately or in a mix – very good)

1. Mix together the soy sauce, vinegar, orange juice, sugar and corn flour.
2. Heat the oil, lard or dripping in a wok or large deep frying pan and fry chicken chunks for 3-4 mins.
3. Add onion, pepper and other vegetables and fry for 4-5 mins till vegetables are tender but still crunchy and the chicken cooked through.
4. Add the sauce and bring to the boil. If too thick add more orange juice or water.
5. Add salt and pepper to taste.

Can be served on a bed of cooked shredded white cabbage, or cooked mashed cauliflower.

Apricot and Nut-stuffed Chicken Breasts

For each person you will need:
- 1 chicken breast
- 4 ready to eat apricots (chopped)
- Small handful of nut (chopped) – cashew, peanuts or almonds
- 1 teaspn. dairy free margarine
- End of a teaspoonful garlic puree
- 1 slice bacon

1. Light oven gas mark 5, 175C, 375F.
2. Grease a baking tray.
3. Mix apricots, nuts, margarine and garlic into a paste.
4. Cut sideways into the chicken breast to make a pocket and put filling inside.
5. Wrap a piece of bacon round the breast to seal the pocket.
6. Bake for 30-35 minutes until cooked through.

This is really delicious and very, very easy to prepare.
Would be nice with green vegetables or salad.

Spiced Turkey Burgers with Guacamole Topping

Serves 4

Burgers:
- 500g or 1 lb. turkey mince
- 2 teasp. harissa paste
- 4 spring onions finely sliced
- 1 tablesp. coriander chopped
- 1 tablesp. chopped mint
- 1 egg yolk
- Freshly ground black pepper

Guacamole:
- 1 avocado, chopped
- 1 medium tomato, finely chopped
- 2 spring onions, finely sliced
- Juice of 1/2 lime

To serve:
- lettuce leaves
- small handful coriander leaves

1. Make the burgers by combining all ingredients and mix well.
2. Wet your hands and shape into 8 patties.
3. Gently fry in oil, lard or dripping till golden and cooked through.
4. Make the guacamole by carefully combining all the ingredients.
5. Lay the burgers on the lettuce leaves and top with the guacamole. Scatter over the coriander leaves.

This is very easy to make.
The burgers will freeze raw or cooked.
Serve with a large mixed salad drizzled with flavored olive oil.

Offal Recipes

Liver, Bacon and Onions

Serves 4

- 600g/ 1lb lamb's liver
- 4 rashers bacon
- 2 large onions
- 2 cloves garlic or 2 teasp. ready garlic from tube
- 1/2 pint beef stock – wheat and dairy free
- Salt and pepper
- 1 level tablesp. Arrowroot or gram flour for thickening

1. Light oven gas 4, 180C, 350 F.
2. Wash the liver in water and slice thinly, removing any tubes or white bits.
3. Place in an oven proof dish with a lid.
4. Peel and slice the onions thinly. Peel and crush the garlic. Layer over the liver.
5. Finely slice the bacon and dry fry in a non-stick frying pan till crisp. Put over the onions.
6. Add the stock, salt and pepper. Put lid on dish and bake in the oven for 3/4 - 1 hour till the liver is tender. Do not overcook as it will go rubbery.
7. To thicken the gravy - NOT for those on Fermenting Gut – mix the arrowroot or gram flour with a little cold water and stir well. Add the hot liquid in the dish to the cold mix, stir well and return to the dish. Put the lid back on and return to the oven for 10 minutes.

Serve with a selection of allowed vegetables.

Beef and Kidney Stew

Serves 4 – 5

- 500g / 1 lb. stewing or braising steak
- 125g / 1/4 lb. lamb's kidneys
- 2 large onions – peeled and chopped
- 2 sticks celery – washed, ends removed and sliced
- 1 courgette – ends removed and chopped into 1-inch cubes
- 1 leek – washed and sliced
- 2 teasp. ready garlic from tube
- 1 large tin chopped tomatoes
- 1 teasp. mixed dried herbs
- 100g mushrooms

1. Light oven 350F, 180 C or gas 4. or use a slow cooker.
2. Cut steak into 1 inch squares. Cut kidneys in half and remove tubes and any white bits. Chop into 1-inch cubes.
3. Put all ingredients into a slow cooker crock or an oven proof casserole with lid.
4. Bake in oven for 2-2 1/2 hours until the meat is tender. Check to see if enough juice is being made from meat and vegetable and add a little water if becoming dry. OR cook in slow cooker for 6-8 hours until the meat is tender, checking the moisture level.
5. For those on the Stone Age Diet (not the Fermenting Gut), you can thicken the gravy with a little gram flour or arrowroot if liked.

Serve with leafy green vegetables and on a bed of shredded cooked white cabbage or cooked mashed cauliflower.

* The stew will freeze.

Cod Ragout

Serves 4

- 2 large leeks
- 2 onions
- 4 carrots
- 2 beef tomatoes (the largest tomatoes you can find)
- 2 tablesp. olive oil, lard or dripping
- Salt
- Black pepper
- 800g or 1 3/4 lbs. cod fillets
- Juice of 1/2 lemon (omit for Fermenting Gut)
- 3 tablesp. olive oil, lard or dripping
- Mild paprika
- Bunch fresh parsley

1. Cut the leeks in half, then into ¼-inch wide strips.
2. Very finely chop the onions and carrots.
3. Skin the tomatoes (pop in boiling water for 1-2 mins. then peel or put on fork and sear over a gas flame then remove skin) and chop the flesh.
4. Put the 2 tablesp. oil, lard or dripping in a large sauce pan. Add leeks, onions and carrots and fry over a low heat for about 10 minutes. Stir often. Add the tomatoes and add salt and pepper to taste. Bring to the boil and then simmer over a low heat.
5. Cut the fish into bite size pieces. Sprinkle with a little salt and the lemon juice. Heat the 3 tablesp. oil, lard or dripping in a frying pan and fry fish for about 3 minutes, turning fish over once. Season with paprika to taste and add fish to the pan of vegetables.
6. Chop the parsley leaves and sprinkle over fish and vegetables.
7. Serve hot.

* This would freeze.

Quick Prawn Curry

Serve 4

- 1 tablesp. oil, lard or dripping
- 1 onion or 3-4 tablesp. ready chopped frozen onion
- 1 -2 teasp. garlic puree
- 2 teasp. chopped ginger - fresh or use ready chopped from a jar
- 1/2-1 teasp. chopped chilies or 1/2 teasp. dried chili flakes
- Large tin chopped tomatoes
- 400g raw peeled prawns
- 2 teasp. garam masala
- 3 tablesp. Kefir or Plain Soya Yogurt
- Handful coriander leaves chopped

1. Heat oil, lard or dripping in pan and gently fry onion, garlic and chili for a few minutes.
2. Add tomatoes and 1 tablesp. water and bring to the boil.
3. Simmer for 2 minutes before adding the prawns and garam masala.
4. Cover and simmer for 5-10 mins.
5. Take off the heat and stir in the yogurt.
6. Sprinkle with coriander.

If you use cooked prawns, only add the prawns right at the end and heat through.
This is simple and easy to make and would taste good with chicken instead of the prawns.
Dice the chicken into small cubes and add the same as the raw prawns but just make sure it is cooked through before serving.
Gram flour pancakes go nicely with this. Poppadum's are also good.
Can be served on a bed of cooked shredded white cabbage, or cooked mashed cauliflower.

Seafood Curry

Serves 4

- 2 tablesp. oil, lard or dripping
- 2 onions chopped
- 1/2 red pepper, deseeded and chopped
- 2 celery sticks chopped
- 1 1/2 teasp. mild curry powder
- 1/2 teasp. turmeric
- 1/2 teasp. ground ginger
- 250g (8oz) haddock fillet diced
- 125 (4 oz.) prawns
- 2 teasp. tomato puree
- 12 tablesp. chicken stock
- Pepper
- 50g (2oz) mushrooms wiped and sliced (Omit for fermenting gut with a yeast problem)
- 1 teasp. Worcestershire sauce
- Juice of half a lemon
- 1 cooking apple, peeled and diced
- 2 tablesp. Soy yogurt or kefir

1. Heat oil, lard or dripping in a large pan. Add the onions, pepper, celery, and mushrooms and fry gently for 5 minutes.
2. Add the curry powder, turmeric, and ginger and cook for a further 2 minutes.
3. Add the apple, haddock, prawns, Worcestershire sauce and tomato puree and stir well. Stir in the stock and season with salt and pepper.
4. Cover and simmer for gently for 10 minutes.
5. Just before serving stir in the lemon juice and the yogurt/kefir.

Serve with green vegetables or on a bed of white cabbage.

Salmon with Herby Roasted Vegetables and Bacon

Serves 2

- 2 x 150g salmon steaks
- 3 small red onions
- 2 teasp. ready garlic
- 2 sticks celery
- 1 red pepper
- 1 green pepper
- 1 courgette
- 2 slices back bacon - diced
- Pinch dried parsley or 2 teasp. chopped fresh parsley
- Pinch salt
- 4-6 tablesp. olive oil, lard or dripping

1. Light oven gas mark 8, 220 C, 450 F.
2. Prepare all vegetables into rough chunks.
3. Put a little oil, lard or dripping in a wok and seal the fish. Remove and keep to one side.
4. Fry bacon in wok till crisp and put into a flat oven proof dish.
5. Put rest of oil, lard or dripping in wok and quickly sear the vegetables. Put oil, lard or dripping and vegetables into the oven proof dish. Add parsley and salt.
6. Roast vegetables in the oven for 1/2 hour.
7. Add the salmon steaks to the vegetables with the skin uppermost.
8. Roast for a further 1/4 hour until the fish is cooked through and the vegetables are soft.
9. Serve.

Ginger and Spring Onion King Prawns

Serves 2

- 225g frozen King Prawns
- 2 spring onions – finely sliced
- 1 teasp. grated fresh ginger or 1 teasp. ready ginger from jar
- 2 tablesp. sesame oil
- 1 teasp. ready garlic from tube

1. Defrost the prawns.
2. Fry spring onions and garlic in very hot oil in a wok or a frying pan for 30 seconds. Stir all the time.
3. Add prawns and ginger and fry on high heat for 1-2 minutes, stirring all the time, till the prawns turn pink. Do not overcook or the prawns will become rubbery.
4. Serve immediately.

This is very good with a vegetable stir fry.

Trout with Prawns

For each person you will need:
- 1 small whole trout
- 50g prawns
- 2 teasp. dairy free spread
- 1 teasp. fresh chopped parsley or 1/2 teasp. dried parsley or herb of your choice

1. Light oven 350 F, 180 C, gas 4.
2. If trout has not been gutted, then slice the fish from the head to the tail down the belly and remove innards.
3. Wash fish under the cold water tap. Lay on a sheet of tin foil large enough to wrap up into a parcel.
4. Mix the herbs with the spread and spread inside the fish.
5. Put the prawns inside the fish. Close the fish up again.
6. Wrap the fish in the foil into a parcel. Place on an oven proof dish and bake for 20-30 minutes until fish is cooked through.

This is very quick and easy to prepare.
This would be good with a mixed tossed salad or roasted vegetables.

Mediterranean Fish Roast

Serve 4

- 2 tablesp. olive oil or sesame seed oil
- 1 large red onion, thinly sliced
- 4 large ripe tomatoes, quartered
- 2 large courgette, trimmed and thinly sliced
- 1 aubergine, trimmed and thinly sliced
- 12 pitted black olives
- 4 skinless white fish fillets – cod, haddock etc. fresh or frozen
- 1 lemon
- 6 tablesp. fish stock or water
- Salt and freshly ground black pepper
- Small handful of roughly chopped fresh parsley to garnish – optional

1. Light oven 200C, 400F, gas 6.
2. Put a little oil in a frying pan and fry the onion till browned and softened.
3. Place all the vegetables in a roasting tin.
4. Arrange the fish on the top of the vegetables.
5. Cut 4 slices from the lemon and place over each piece of fish.
6. Squeeze the juice from the rest of the lemon and drizzle over the fish. Add the stock or the water and drizzle with the olive oil.
7. Roast for 20 minutes or until the fish is cooked through and the vegetables are soft.
8. Sprinkle with salt and pepper and scatter over the parsley.

Serve with green vegetables.
This is quick and easy to prepare and cook.

Roasted Spiced Cod

Serves 4

- 1 lemon or 2-3 tablesp. ready lemon juice from bottle
- 2 teasp. mild curry powder
- 4 X 200g chunky cod fillet
- 1 tablesp. olive oil

1. Light oven 200C, gas mark 6.
2. Place fish on a non-stick baking sheet.
3. Sprinkle over the lemon juice and the curry powder, and drizzle with olive oil.
4. Bake for 10 minutes 'til fish is cooked through.
5. Serve hot.

This would be good with a large mixed salad or cooked vegetables like green beans, cauliflower, broccoli and carrots.

Tandoori Prawn Skewers

Serves 4

- 300g raw peeled king prawns – washed
- 2 tablesp. tomato puree
- 2 tablesp. kefir
- 1/2 teasp. mild chili powder
- 1 teasp. garam masala
- 1 teasp. ground cumin
- 2 teasp. coriander seeds crushed or 1 teasp. coriander powder

1. Mix prawns with all ingredients and leave to marinate overnight or for at least 2 hours.
2. Soak wooden skewers in water for 30 minutes, then thread 3 prawns on each skewer.
3. Either grill on BBQ for 1-2 minutes each side or heat a griddle pan or a non- stick frying pan and cook for 1-2 minutes on each side.
4. Serve hot.

This would be good with a salad in warm weather or roasted vegetables in cold weather.

Thai Steamed Salmon

Serves 4

- 4 salmon fillets (skinned)
- 1 small bunch coriander (chopped including stalks)
- 12 mint leaves (chopped)
- 12 Thai basil leaves (chopped)
- 2 cloves garlic (crushed)
- 3 tablesp. fresh lime juice
- 1 inch fresh ginger (grated)
- 1 tablesp. fish sauce (Nam Pla)
- 2 green chilies deseeded and chopped (opt)

1. Whizz all the ingredients (except salmon) in a food processor to a smoothish paste.
2. Pour over the salmon and marinate for 30 mins (or more).
3. Steam the salmon in a bowl with the marinade for 10 mins.
4. Serve with steamed bok choi or other greens.

There will be plenty of sauce remaining to pour over.

Fish Burgers

Serves 4

- 500g fish (skinned, boned and cubed)
- 2 tablesp. red onion (finely chopped)
- Zest of 1/2 lemon
- 1 tablesp. capers (drained and rinsed)
- 1-2 tablesp. parsley (finely chopped)
- Large pinch of salt

1. Whizz half the fish to a paste in a food processor.
2. Add the remaining ingredients and pulse until combined and you have a rough mix.
3. Shape into burgers and fry for 2-4 minutes (depending on thickness) each side.

Seared/Roasted Halibut

Serves 4

- 1 orange, juiced
- 3 tablesp. coconut aminos
- 2 tablesp. lemon juice
- 1/2 teasp. ginger powder
- 1/2 teasp. sea salt
- 2 tablesp. coconut flour
- 3 tablesp. coconut oil
- 4x halibut fillets
- 1.5-2" thick skinned chives for garnishing

1. Preheat your oven to 200C degrees.
2. Combine the orange juice, coconut aminos, lemon juice, ginger and half the sea salt in a small bowl, set aside.
3. Spread the coconut flour on a plate.
4. Dry the fish with kitchen towel.
5. Sprinkle both sides with the remaining sea salt and place in the coconut flour, making sure it's all coated.
6. Heat the coconut oil in an oven-safe frying pan on medium-high heat. When very hot, add the halibut and sear for a minute or so on one side, until browned. Turn and place immediately in the top of the oven.
7. Cook for 5-10 minutes (depending on the thickness of your fillet) until the fish is opaque.
8. Place fish on warmed plates and pour the sauce mixture into the hot pan. Allow to bubble for a minute and then pour over the fish.
9. Garnish with fresh chopped chives.

Serve with greens and any allowed vegetables of your choice.

Grilled Sesame Salmon with Rocket Salad

Serves 4

- 4 x 200g thick salmon fillets
- 4 tablesp. sesame oil
- 4 teasp. sesame seeds
- 2 ripe and ready avocadoes
- 200g cherry tomatoes
- 75 rocket leaves
- 1 tablesp. lemon juice
- 2 tablesp. olive oil
- 40g toasted pine nuts

1. Preheat the grill and put salmon onto a lined grill pan. Brush salmon on both sides with sesame oil and press on the sesame seeds.
2. Grill for 10 minutes turning once till cooked through.
3. Quarter the avocadoes, remove stones, peel away the skin and slice.
4. Divide the avocadoes, tomatoes and rocket leaves between 4 plates.
5. Shake together the lemon juice and olive oil and drizzle over the salad.
6. Place hot salmon on top and sprinkle with toasted pine nuts.

Vegetable Recipes

Ratatouille

Serves 4

- 1 Aubergine chopped into small cubes
- 1 onion or 3-4 tablesp. ready chopped frozen onion
- 2 courgette
- any other vegetables you have to hand like mange tout, green beans etc.
- 1 large tin chopped tomatoes
- 1 stock cube (dairy free and wheat free)
- 1 teasp. dried herbs or 1 tablesp. fresh herbs like coriander or rosemary
- salt and pepper
- large handful mushrooms sliced or 1 small tin ready sliced mushrooms (omit for Fermenting Gut with a yeast problem)

1. Put all chopped and sliced vegetables into a saucepan with the stock cube, tomatoes and herbs. Do not add any water as the water will come out of the vegetables. Add salt and pepper to taste.
2. Bring to the boil, then simmer for 30-40 minutes (with a lid on the pan) till all the vegetable are soft and pulpy.

This will freeze or keep in the fridge for a few days and is good to eat with „dry" meats like chops or chicken breasts instead of gravy. Wheat free sausages can be fried, chopped and added to the ratatouille to make a tasty sausage stew.

Tomato Salsa

- 1 small red onion
- 1 spring onion
- 1/2 red pepper
- 1/2 green pepper
- 1 stick celery
- 300g large tomatoes
- 50g sun dried tomatoes in oil
- 20ml basil flavored olive oil
- 30 ml olive oil
- pinch dried oregano
- 1/2 teasp. Paprika pepper
- 20g tomato puree
- For a hot salsa add chili to taste

1. Very finely chop all vegetables. Use a hand chopper or a food processor.
2. Combine all ingredients. Mix well.
3. Divide in half and blend one half till pureed.
4. Combine with the other half and mix well.
5. Store in a sealed container in the fridge.

This is delicious with burgers, sausages, chicken, chops etc. or just serve over a salad as a dressing.

Cauliflower with Tomatoes and Cumin

Serves 4

- 2 tablesp. sunflower or olive oil, lard or dripping
- 1 onion chopped
- 1 teasp. ready garlic from tube
- 1 small cauliflower broken into florets
- 1 teasp. cumin seeds
- a good pinch ground ginger
- 1 small tin or 1/2 large tin tomatoes
- 2 tablesp. chopped coriander
- salt and freshly ground black pepper
- 1-2 teasp. lemon juice

1. Heat the oil, lard or dripping in a large pan. Add the onions and garlic and fry gently for 2-3 minutes until the onion is softened.
2. Add the cauliflower and fry for a further 2-3 minutes until the cauliflower is flecked with brown. Add the cumin seeds and ginger and fry briskly for 1 minute, then add the tomatoes, 175 ml / 6 fl. oz. water and salt and pepper. Cover the pan with a lid.
3. Bring to the boil and then reduce heat and simmer for 6-7 minutes till the cauliflower is just cooked. Do not overcook the cauliflower as it will just turn to mush.
4. Stir in the lemon juice (if allowed), scatter over the coriander and serve at once.

This would be good with chicken, fish or pork cooked in the oven or on the BBQ with extra vegetables or a large mixed salad.

Asparagus and Bacon Stir Fry

Serves 2

- 100g fresh asparagus – cut into inch lengths
- 2 rashers bacon – finely sliced
- 2 spring onions – finely sliced
- 1 stick celery – finely sliced
- 1 red pepper – de-seeded and finely sliced or equivalent in frozen peppers
- 1 courgette – finely sliced or diced
- 1/2 packet bean sprouts or 1 tin bean sprouts – drained
- 2 teasp. ready garlic from tube
- 3 tablesp. any flavor oil, lard or dripping

1. Boil cut asparagus in water for 5 minutes. Drain.
2. Fry bacon and garlic in the very hot oil, lard or dripping for 3 minutes on high heat, tossing all the time.
3. Add onions, celery, pepper and courgette and fry on high heat, tossing all the time, for 2 minutes.
4. Add asparagus and bean sprouts and fry on high heat, tossing all the time, for a further 2 minutes.
5. Serve hot.

This goes well with Ginger and Spring Onion King Prawns or any meat such as burgers, chops, chicken breast etc.

Courgettes with Moroccan Spices

Serves 4

- 500g / 1 1/4 lb. courgette
- Chopped fresh coriander and parsley to serve

For the spicy charmoula:
- 1 onion – finely chopped
- 2 teasp. ready garlic from tube
- 1/4 red or green chili – de-seeded and finely sliced
- 1/2 teasp. paprika pepper
- 1/2 ground cumin
- 3 tablesp. olive oil
- salt and freshly ground black pepper

1. Light oven 180C, 350F, gas 4.
2. Take the ends off the courgette and slice lengthways into quarters or eighths, depending on their thickness. Place in a shallow oven proof dish or casserole.
3. Mix all the ingredients for the charmoula with 4 tablesp. cold water. Pour over courgette. Cover with a lid and cook for 15 minutes till the courgette are soft.

This would be good served with chicken breasts, white fish or pork chops cooked in the oven (put in oven before courgette to allow time to cook through) and on a bed of cooked shredded white cabbage or cooked mashed cauliflower.

Deep Fried Spinach

Serve 3-4

- 1 large pack of baby spinach leaves ready washed and dried
- Oil for deep frying

1. Heat the oil in a deep pan.
2. Fry a large handful of spinach in the oil for a few moments till shriveled and crispy. Remove from oil into a hot dish lined with kitchen roll. Keep hot.
3. Repeat the frying till all the spinach is used up.
4 Serve hot.

It's like crispy seaweed and is really good with Chinese style dishes. This is really great to put on top of stir fries.

Roasted Vegetables

- Selection of allowed vegetables such as carrots, onions, cherry tomatoes, celery, courgette, green beans, sugar snap peas, leeks, garlic cloves, aubergines, sun dried tomatoes etc.
- 2 tablesp. per person oil – olive, herb, coconut, sesame or lemon oils
- 1 teasp. dried mixed herbs

1. Light oven 200C, 400F, gas mark 6.
2. Peel and prepare vegetables, making sure they are the same size chunks.
3. Put into oven proof dish and cover with oil, add a small amount of water.
4. Sprinkle over herbs and bake in oven for approximately 45 minutes until vegetables are soft and golden brown.

You can add chicken breasts or fish on top of the vegetables.
For chicken, add after 15 minutes and cook for a further 30 minutes or until the chicken is cooked through.
For fish, add after 30 minutes and cook for a further 15 minutes till fish is cooked through.
If any vegetables left over, they can whizzed up with stock and /or tomato passata to make a great tasty soup.

Sauerkraut

- 1kg grated veg (cabbage/carrot etc)
- 25g grated ginger (optional)
- 1 tablesp. sea salt

(Multiply above as needed.)

1. Mix all the ingredients in a bowl, pummel/kneed/squeeze the mix until liquid appears.
2. Transfer to sterilized kilner jars and pack in as tightly as possible (leave about 1 cm gap at the top). If the liquid doesn't cover the veg; leave the lids down, but not sealed, place somewhere tepid and out of direct sunlight for 24 hours. (Every now and then give the kraut a squidge to encourage liquid production.)
3. After 24 hours if the veg is still not covered by liquid mix 1 teasp. salt with 1 cup of water and add enough to cover the kraut.
4. Seal the lids tightly and leave to ferment for another 6-7 days (longer the better). Once you begin to eat store in the fridge.

Fresher veg produces liquid faster.

Roasted Garlic and Lemon Cauliflower

Serves 4

- 1 large head of cauliflower (cut into florets)
- 1/4 cup of lard, ghee, tallow or coconut oil
- 8-10 cloves fresh garlic, crushed
- Zest of 1 lemon
- 1/4 teasp. salt
- 1/4 teasp. pepper
- handful chopped fresh parsley

1. Preheat oven to 220C.
2. Melt cooking fat in a casserole over a medium heat.
3. Add all the ingredients (except parsley) and toss in the oil.
4. Place the lid on the casserole and roast for 25-35 minutes (depending on how big your florets are) stirring once halfway through.
5. Remove from oven and toss with fresh parsley.

This can be served with any main meal.

Courgette Pasta with Bacon

Serves 4

- 4 large courgette
- 2 teasp. salt
- 1 teasp. avocado oil
- 200g pancetta cubes or bacon bits
- 1/4 cup chopped fresh basil
- 2 large garlic cloves, crushed
- 1/2 cup chopped Walnuts (optional)

1. Finely julienne the courgette lengthwise to create long strips of courgette. Toss with salt in a colander and let sit in the sink for 1 hour.
2. Rinse the courgette very, very thoroughly (have a taste to make sure it's not salty at all). Drain on a tea towel or paper towels to get rid of as much moisture as possible.
3. Heat the oil in an oversized frying pan over medium-high heat. Add the bacon and cook until golden brown and some of the fat has been released. Add garlic & courgette, turn the heat up a little and sauté, stirring frequently until the courgette just begins to soften (4-5 minutes).
4. Toss in basil and walnuts (if using) and cook for another minute or so, stirring a couple of times.

Roasted Butternut Squash

- 1 large butternut squash, peeled, seeded and cut into 1 1/2" pieces
- 2 tablesp. extra virgin coconut oil or other oil of choice
- 2 teasp. fresh thyme, chopped (or dried thyme)
- 1 teasp. sea salt

1. Preheat oven to 200C, gas mark 6.
2. Put the oil in a large roasting tin and place in the oven to melt.
3. Add the other ingredients to the pan and toss in the oil.
4. Bake for 30-35 minutes, giving the squash a toss halfway through, until slightly browned and tender.

Oven Roast Cauliflower and Broccoli with Garlic

Serves up to 4

- 8 oz. cauliflower
- 8 oz. Broccoli
- 2 garlic cloves peeled and chopped
- 1 heaped teasp. whole coriander seed coarsely crushed
- 2 teasp. olive oil
- Salt and pepper to taste

1. Pre heat oven to gas mark 6, 400 F.
2. Trim the cauliflower and broccoli into floret. Place in a mixing bowl then sprinkle with crushed coriander seeds, garlic and olive oil.
3. Toss the mix gently then arrange the mix into a roasting tin.
4. Place in the oven for 30 minutes.

Bean Filling for Stuffed Marrow, Courgette or Green Pepper

Serves 2-3

- 1 onion
- 1 green, orange or red pepper
- few mushrooms
- large tin red kidney beans
- 1-2 tablesp. oil
- mixed herbs

1. Light oven: Gas Mark 5, 190C, 375F.
2. Cut chosen vegetable to be stuffed in half lengthways and remove seeds.
3. Chop other vegetables.
4. Fry in oil till softened and golden brown.
5. Add large pinch herbs and drained beans.
6. Stir till hot.
7. Place chosen vegetable in oven proof dish and fill with bean mixture.
8. Drizzle a little olive oil over the vegetables and bake till tender.

Coleslaw

- 1/4 white cabbage
- 1/8 red cabbage(opt)
- 2 carrots
- Wheat free and dairy free mayonnaise (Plamil)
- Chopped nuts and /or seeds can be added

1. Peel the carrots and grate.
2. Shred the cabbage finely and put in a large bowl.
3. Add enough mayonnaise to bind together.
4. Taste and add salt and pepper if liked.

* This will store, covered, in the fridge overnight.

Chickpea and Spinach Curry

Serves 4

- 1 1/2 teasp. ready chopped ginger
- 1-2 teasp. ready red chilies
- 400g tin chopped tomatoes
- 450g spinach leaves
- 600g tinned chickpeas, drained and rinsed
- 200g frozen diced onion or 2 medium onions chopped
- 2 teasp. garlic puree
- 2 tablesp. mild or medium curry powder or paste (depending on how hot you like curry)

1. Spray a large saucepan or wok with low-calorie cooking spray. Add onions, garlic and ginger and cook for 5 mins till softened and golden.
2. Add curry powder and chilies and cook gently for 3 mins.
3. Add tomatoes and spinach and simmer for 5 mins.
4. Add chick peas and continue to simmer for 5-10 mins. Add salt and pepper to taste.

Can be served on a bed of cooked shredded white cabbage, or cooked mashed cauliflower
This can be made, kept in the fridge and microwaved when needed.
Gram flour pancakes go nicely with this. Poppadum's are also good.

Desserts and Puddings

Easy Chocolate Mousse

Serves 8-10 in small portions

- 1 carton silken tofu
- 4 tablesp. xylitol or other allowed sweetener (or to taste)
- 4 tablesp. raw cacao powder or Green & Blacks cocoa powder (or to taste)
- Splash vanilla essence

1. Place all ingredients into a blender or food processor.
2. Blend until well combined.
3. Taste, and adjust composition if necessary.
4. Refrigerate in a pretty bowl or individual dishes (shot glasses are also fun!).

This is very rich, so keep your portion sizes small. I have served this to many, many people, and none of them guessed this was not only sugar-free but also vegan!
You can use different flavors too, but I find the cocoa nicely masks the bland, slightly savory taste of the tofu.

Chocolate Pudding

Serves 4

- 2 avocados
- 2 desert spoons of cocoa powder (or raw cacao)
- 1 teaspn to 2 tablesp. coconut oil (optional - depending on how rich you want it)
- 1-2 teasp. lecithin (optional)
- Xylitol (according to taste)

1. Just whizz up all ingredients in a blender or food processor.
2. Pour into individual dishes or one bowl.

Can substitute half cocoa powder with carob if allowed (I substitute half cocoa with white Peruvian carob which is OK for candida maintenance diets and lower GI than ordinary carob).
Can substitute xylitol with d-ribose or a different allowed sweetener. I decorate the top with a few raw cacao nibs.
Kefir (or coconut milk or allowed milk substitute) can be added to make a chocolate Kefir delight.

Apple and Coconut Omelet

Serves 1

- 1 tablesp. coconut oil
- 2 eggs
- One peeled and sliced apple with a dash of cinnamon
- 1 tablesp. desiccated coconut for added fiber

1. Heat oil in small frying pan and gently fry apple slices till soft.
2. Beat eggs together, add desiccated coconut and add to pan. Allow eggs to set while gently pulling cooked egg away from sides of pan.
3. If liked, the top can be grilled to a light brown colour.
4. Serve at once.

Instant Hot Chocolate Almond Sponge Cake

Serves 1

- 4 good tablesp. of ground almond flour
- 1 small egg.
- 1/4 teaspoon of bicarbonate of soda
- 1 good teaspoon of cocoa

1. Mix all ingredients well in a mug, then microwave on 800w for 40 seconds.
2. Take it out and give it a poke so it doesn't stick to sides then microwave for another 40 seconds.
3. It should look like a small sponge cake / dumpling.

If you microwave it for too long will end up a bit chewy.
Serve with dark chocolate melted on the top, kefir and berries.
You can add different ingredients depending on what you can tolerate, nuts, seeds, stevia, grated carrot or mixed herbs without the cocoa for a savory dish. It's very, very filling.
You can also make one and it will keep for a couple of days in fridge to slice and toast.

Faux Yo

Serves 1

- 4 tablesp. soy kefir
- 3 tablesp. Blue Dragon coconut cream (note: this is NOT the same as creamed coconut)

1. Mix the ingredients together.
2. Use as you would yogurt, e.g. add berries, nuts, hemp seeds, etc.

This is a very palatable way to eat both components – the coconut cream takes the tangy edge off the kefir and adds a creamy sweetness, whilst the kefir tempers the richness of the coconut cream.

Stone Age "Ice Cream"

Serves 6-8

- 1 400ml can coconut milk, shaken
- 3-4 tablesp. xylitol or other permitted sweetener (to taste)
- 2 fresh egg yolks
- Flavoring of your choosing (see below)

1. Place the egg yolks in a large jug and whisk briefly with a hand held whisk to break up (they do not need to become fluffy or anything).
2. Mix the coconut milk and xylitol together in a saucepan. Heat gently until warm, stirring frequently.
3. Temper the egg yolks by adding one small ladleful of the warm milk mixture at a time and whisking constantly.
4. Once all the milk has been added to the yolks and is well mixed, add your preferred flavoring from list „A" and leave to cool. Once cool, place in the fridge to chill.
5. Use a budget ice cream maker to churn your "ice cream", adding ingredients from list „B" towards the end or sprinkling on top. Alternatively, freeze the mixture in a shallow dish, stirring regularly to break up any large ice crystals.
6. Either enjoy straightaway OR freeze in a plastic container for later.

List A (ingredients to add at the mixing/whisking stage):
vanilla extract, peppermint extract, cacao powder, lemon extract, espresso decaffeinated coffee, cinnamon, nutmeg, mixed spice, cacao powder & cayenne pepper

List B (ingredients to add near the end of churning or to sprinkle on top): desiccated coconut, toasted almonds, high cocoa chocolate drops, cacao nibs, roasted walnuts, chopped hazelnuts, lemon zest, orange zest, blanched almonds, your choice of berries.

I Can't Believe It's Not Ice Cream

- 2 cups of sunflower oil (or rape seed oil or hemp oil)
- 1 cup of soya milk (or coconut milk, rice milk, almond milk)
- 1/4 teaspn. liquid lecithin (can be soya or sunflower)
- 5 g of D ribose
- 1 teaspoon vanilla essence

1. Whizz up in smoothie maker or blender.
2. If too runny, add more oil. If too thick, add more liquid.
3. Add frozen berries to the smoothie mix – this breaks up the berries and the mix freezes solid as ice cream as it stirs.

If it does not freeze when the berries are added, then put the mixture in plastic container with lid and put in the freezer.
Keep in the freezer.

Chocolate Nut Torte

Equipment: You need a food processor.
I usually use a 9-inch spring-form pan, but you could use e.g. 12 muffin tins.

Base:
- 1 rounded tablesp. goji berries
- 1 cup whole almonds
- 1/3 cup cocoa powder
- 2 tablesp. xylitol
- 1 teasp. vanilla

Filling:
- 2 cups raw cashews, soaked overnight and rinsed
- 1/2 cup water
- 1/4 cup xylitol, with water added to just cover (i.e. up to 1/4 cup mark)
- 1/4 teasp. salt
- 1/4 cup + 2 tablesp. almond butter or peanut butter
- 1 1/2 cup coconut oil, melted
- 1/2 cup cocoa powder
- 1 pinch sea salt

Base:
1. Put the goji berries into a small dish or cup and add water to just cover the berries. Leave to soften for about 15-20 minutes.
2. Line the bottom of the spring-form pan with baking parchment.
3. Put the almonds into the processor and whizz until chopped into medium / small pieces.
4. Add cocoa powder, xylitol, vanilla, salt and the goji berries, together with the soaking liquid.
5. Process again. The mixture should begin to hold together – if it doesn't, add a drop more water.
6. Press the mixture into the bottom of the pan.
7. Set aside while you making the filling.
8. I often have a rest at this point

Filling:
1. Put drained cashews, water, xylitol & liquid and salt into the processor. Blend until really smooth, scraping down the sides of the processor as necessary.
2. Add cocoa powder and nut butter to the cashew mixture and blend all together; then pour in the melted coconut oil, and process until completely mixed.
3. Spread the filling onto the base.
4. Put the torte into the freezer until solid (about 3 hours for large torte).
5. Remove torte from pan and cut into slices (about 14). If it's too hard to cut, leave for a while until a little softer. Store slices in freezer until required.

To serve – remove from freezer about 30 minutes before required, to allow the torte to soften before eating. It's a rich torte – but very yummy!

Chocolate Mousse

Serves 4-6

Mousse:
- 4 ounces 71%+ cacao dark chocolate
- 3 ounces filtered water
- pinch sea salt
- few drops orange extract (optional)
- 1-2 ice cube trays worth of ice

Whipped Cream:
- 1/2 can coconut milk (refrigerated)
- 1/4 teasp vanilla or almond extract

Garnish:
- coarse sea salt

1. Simply pour water into a saucepan. Then, over medium-low heat, whisk in the chocolate. The result is a homogenous sauce.
2. Put the saucepan in a bowl partly filled with ice cubes (or pour into another bowl over the ice - it will chill faster), then whisk the chocolate sauce, either manually with a whisk or with an electric mixer (if using an electric mixer, watch closely - it will thicken faster). Whisking creates large air bubbles in the sauce, which steadily thickens. After a while strands of chocolate form inside the loops of the whisk. Pour or spoon immediately into ramekins, small bowls or jars and let set.
3. Note: Three things can go wrong. Here's how to fix them. If your chocolate doesn't contain enough fat, melt the mixture again, add some more chocolate, and then whisk it again. If the mousse is not light enough, melt the mixture again, add some water, and whisk it once more. If you whisk it too much, so that it becomes grainy, this means that the foam has turned into an emulsion. In that case simply melt the mixture and whisk it again, adding nothing.
4. Serve immediately, or refrigerate.

If you're making whipped cream:
1. Remove your bowl and beater from the freezer.
2. Turn the can of coconut milk upside down and open the bottom. Spoon half the thickened, chilled coconut milk into the mixing bowl and save the rest for a curry.
3 Add the extract to the bowl, then beat the coconut milk for 5 or so minutes until it takes on the texture of whipped cream.
4. Dollop on top of the mousse, then sprinkle the top of the dessert with a pinch of coarse sea salt.
5. Serve and relish the compliments.

Raspberry Panna Cotta

Serves 4 - 6 depending on serving size

Panna Cotta
- 2 cups full-fat coconut milk
- 1/4 cup fresh lemon juice
- 2 teasp. gelatin
- 2 tablesp. xylitol or Truvia
- 250g raspberries
- Pinch sea salt

Raspberry Sauce
- 125g raspberries
- 1 tablesp. xylitol or truvia
- 1/2 teasp. vanilla extract

For the Panna Cotta:

1. Squeeze the lemon juice into a small shallow/wide bowl. Sprinkle the gelatin over the top and leave to bloom for a few minutes.
2. In a small pan over a low heat add 1/2 cup of the coconut milk. Once beginning to warm add the sweetener and the gelatin mix. Whisk until all combined and smooth.
3. Pour into a blender with the remaining coconut milk and raspberries. Blend until smooth.
4. Pour this mixture in batches through a fine sieve to remove the seeds. You will need to push it through with a wooden spoon or spatula.
5. Divide between serving bowls/glasses and chill in the fridge for 2+ hours.

For the sauce:
1. Heat all the ingredients in a small saucepan over a medium/low heat. Squish the berries with a spoon as they heat.
2. Once it begins to bubble remove from the heat and pass through a fine sieve to remove the seeds.

3. Refrigerate until ready to serve - pour over Panna Cottas when ready.

Bread Substitute Recipes

American Pancakes

Makes 4 x 5-6 inch pancakes

- 3/4 cup gram flour (chick pea or garbanzo bean flour)
- 1/4 cup tapioca or oat flour
- 2 heaped teasp. baking Powder (wheat free)
- 2 tablesp. olive oil
- Approx. 1 cup water

1. Place all dry ingredients into a bowl. Stir.
2. Add the oil and enough water to make a batter which will coat the back of a spoon. This will
probably thicken up while standing and you may need to thin it down.
3. Heat a griddle or non- stick frying pan till hot.
4. Pour out batter to make a 5-6-inch circle on the griddle – a quarter of the mixture. You may have room for more than one.
5. Allow to cook till the surface is well bubbled, the pancake well risen and looks nearly cooked – no runny mixture – about 4 - 5 minutes. It will be slightly brown underneath. Turn over pancake and cook for a further 1-2 minutes. These can be kept hot in a warm oven on kitchen paper on a baking sheet till all have been cooked.
6. Serve with non-dairy spread and very crispy streaky bacon.

Yummie!

Savory Gram (Chick Pea) Flour Pancakes

Makes 4 large pancakes

- 100g/4oz chickpea flour (gram)
- 1/2 teasp. salt
- 1/2 teasp. cayenne pepper opt.
- Black Pepper
- 330ml/11 fl. oz. water
- Oil for frying

1. Preheat the oven to very low. In a large mixing bowl, mix together the flour, salt, cayenne and Black pepper.
2. Gradually add the water, beating well, until you get a smooth batter. Add a little more water if necessary.
3. Heat a little oil in a non-stick frying pan, add a quarter of the batter, swirling it around the base to coat evenly, and cook until the edges are crispy and brown, and the top has dried out.
4. Turn the pancake and cook for another minute till browned on that side. Transfer to a warm plate, cover loosely with foil and keep warm in the oven whilst you cook the remaining pancakes.
5. Serve with the savory or „sweet" filling of your choice.

These are very good.
Can be used as wraps.
Better hot.

Yorkshire Oatcakes

Makes 6-7 small oatcakes. Serves 2.

This traditional Yorkshire recipe has been adapted for the Stone Age Diet by using oat flour instead of ordinary flour and wheat free baking powder.

- 3 oz. / 75gm fine oatmeal
- 1 oz. / 25gm oat flour
- 1 tablesp. olive oil
- 1/4 pint / 150ml water
- 1 heaped teasp. wheat free baking powder
- large pinch salt

1. Mix all ingredients together till smooth.
2. Heat a griddle or a large non-stick frying pan. Lightly rub some oil over or use 1 cal. spray oil.
3. Drop 1 tablesp. of the mixture onto the pan/griddle for each oatcake until pan is full. Leave enough space for oatcakes to spread without running into one another. Cook on medium heat, 3- 4 minutes, till cake is bubbly and looks cooked - not still waxy. Turn oatcake over and cook for 1-2 minutes. The cakes will brown very slightly.
4. Place cooked oatcakes in a folded cloth to keep hot and cook remaining mixture after greasing the pan again.

Eat hot with dairy free margarine. These make a good substitute for bread and are particularly good with Home Made Soups.
Any leftover oatcakes can be cooled, put in a plastic bag and reheated the next day either in the microwave or in the toaster.
They will also freeze so you could double the mixture and have a ready supply in the freezer.

Wheat-free Rosemary-Thyme Crackers

Makes about 20 crackers

- 1 1/2 cups blanched almond flour
- 2 tablesp. ground flax seed
- 1 tablesp. fresh rosemary + 1 tablesp. fresh thyme, finely chopped
- 1/2 teasp. fine sea salt
- 1/8 teasp. freshly ground black pepper
- 1 tablesp. olive oil
- 1 egg
- 2 teaspoons water

1. Preheat the oven to 350. In a small bowl, lightly whisk the oil, egg and water to combine. In a larger bowl, combine the rest of the ingredients into a uniform dry mixture.
2. Add the wet ingredients to the dry ingredients and stir well to combine. Once the dough comes together, use your clean hands to mix well and ensure a uniform mixture.
3. Place the dough between two sheets of parchment paper and roll out to 1/8-inch thickness. Peel off the top sheet of parchment paper and place the bottom sheet with dough onto baking sheet.
4. Cut into 2-inch squares and bake 12-15 minutes until lightly golden around the edges. Let cool at least 15 minutes before serving.
5. Store in the refrigerator up to one week, or at room temperature up to two days.

Cook's notes:
I live in a very dry climate. If you're in a more humid climate, you may not need to add the 2 teaspoons of water.
Thin dough (1/8 inch) makes crispier crackers; thicker dough (1/4 inch) makes softer, chewier crackers.
I used rosemary and thyme here, but two tablesp. of any combination of fresh finely chopped herbs can be used.

Flax Seed (Linseed) Loaf

- 100g flax meal – very finely ground
- 20g ground almonds
- half a teaspoon of salt
- half a teaspoon of bicarbonate of soda

Plus, optional to taste:
- cinnamon or
- cardamom or
- cumin seeds/powder or
- finely grated courgette or
- finely grated lemon rind or
- oregano (or other herbs & spices)
- 2 eggs
- one third of a cup (approx. 80-90ml) of water or kefir
- one third of a cup of olive (or sunflower) oil

1. Light oven gas 2, 150 C, 300 F.
2. Grease and line with grease proof paper a 1lb. loaf tin.
3. Mix together the dry ingredients.
4. In a separate bowl, mix together the wet ingredients.
5. Then add the dry ingredients to the wet mixture and mix together well.
6. Put mixture into loaf tin and bake for 50-60 minutes.
7. Remove from oven, leave to cool for 5 minutes then take loaf out of tin, remove paper and cool on a wire rack.

Refrigerate if you intend keeping it for more than 1-2 days.
This is good spread with dairy free spread.
Can be served instead of bread or any carbohydrate usually served with a main meal.

Low-carb Ground Almond Slice

Makes about 16 slices

- 5 cups (500g or 1 lb.) ground almond flour
- 1 teasp. sea salt
- 1 teasp. bicarbonate of soda
- 1 1/2 cups (340g or 12 oz.) of pure dairy free spread or Vitalite or other non- dairy butter
- 4 Free Range Eggs or ordinary eggs

1. Light oven gas 2, 150 C, 300 F.
2. Grease a baking sheet or use a non - stick baking sheet.
3. Mix dry ingredients together (almond flour, salt and bicarbonate of soda).
4. Mix wet ingredients together with electric whisk (dairy free spread and eggs).
5. Stir wet ingredients into dry with wooden spoon, until a sticky mixture is formed (dough-like).
6. Take a small hand full of mixture, roll into a ball, then flatten between hands (should make about 16).
7. Lay on a greased or non - stick baking tray.
8. Bake for about one hour or until turning golden brown. Obviously the longer you cook them, the harder they will be.
9. Leave to cool then store in fridge.

You can:
- toast them
- eat fresh from the fridge
- or, my favorite, warmed in microwave for about 15 - 20 seconds, then served with raspberries, blueberries and ice cold coconut kefir.

If you are feeling naughty, you can warm it up with one square of 85% dark chocolate, it's really filling.
Useful for spreading things on!

Broccoli Bread

- Makes 1 loaf
- 1 broccoli head (remove most of the stalk) steamed or boiled till soft
- 1/2 cup ground almonds
- 1/2 cup gram flour
- 2 teasp. Bicarbonate of Soda
- 1/2 cup egg white
- 2 whole eggs
- 1/2 cup soya milk

1. Light oven 160C, 300F, gas mark 2.
2. Mix all powdered ingredients in a bowl.
3. Add eggs, whites and milk, add cooked broccoli and blend all together with a blender to a smooth consistency.
4. Pour into a greased and lined bread tin and bake for 40-60 minutes till the top springs back when pressed lightly.
5. Allow to cool in the tin, before turning out.

Slice cold.
This can be eaten as it is or toasted and served hot.
This will freeze, sliced.

Dressings

Tomato Salsa

- 1 small red onion
- 1 spring onion
- 1/2 red pepper
- 1/2 green pepper
- 1 stick celery
- 300g large tomatoes
- 50g sun dried tomatoes in oil
- 20ml basil flavored olive oil
- 30 ml olive oil
- pinch dried oregano
- 1/2 teasp. Paprika pepper
- 20g tomato puree
- For a hot salsa add chili to taste

1. Very finely chop all vegetables. Use a hand chopper or a food processor.
2. Combine all ingredients. Mix well.
3. Divide in half and blend one half till pureed.
4. Combine with the other half and mix well.
5. Store in a sealed container in the fridge.

This is delicious with burgers, sausages, chicken, chops etc. or just serve over a salad as a dressing.

Garlic Mayonnaise

- 2-3 garlic cloves peeled or 2-3 teasp. ready garlic in tube
- 10oz /290g pack of silken tofu
- 180ml / 6fl oz. / 3/4 cup of sunflower oil
- Salt and pepper to taste

1. Crush the garlic cloves and process with the tofu until smooth
2. Gradually add the sunflower oil with food processor on full power until the ingredients are well combined
3. Season with salt and pepper.
4. Refrigerate and use with 3 days

Lemon Vinaigrette

- 1 cup olive oil
- 1/2 cup lemon juice
- Salt and freshly ground black pepper to taste

1. Put all ingredients into a screw top jar and shake well.

Always shake the jar before pouring to mix the oil and lemon juice. This keeps well in the fridge for at least a couple of weeks.

French Dressing

- 8 tablesp. virgin olive oil
- 4 tablesp. lemon juice
- 1 level teasp. dried mustard powder
- Salt and freshly ground black pepper

1. Put all ingredients into a screw topped jar and shake well.

This will keep for 3-4 weeks in the fridge.
The dressing needs to be shaken each time it is poured.

Mayonnaise

- 2 cups of olive oil (or sunflower oil, rape seed oil or hemp oil)
- 1 cup of soya milk (or coconut milk, rice milk, almond milk)
- Lemon juice, garlic, mustard, salt – to taste
- 1/2 teaspoon of lecithin to emulsify

1. Whizz up in food processor or smoothie maker.

Store in a screw top jar.

Lasts several days in the fridge.

Sweet Mustard Salad Dressing

This makes enough for 2-3 servings. For a full bottle multiply recipe by 7.

- 2 tablesp. olive oil
- 1 tablesp. cider vinegar or lemon juice
- 8-10 drops Stevia or more if you like it sweeter
- 1 level teasp. dried mustard
- 1 level teasp. white mustard seeds
- pinch salt
- freshly ground black pepper

1. Put all ingredients in a screw top jar and shake well.

Always shake bottle well before pouring to mix the oil in.
This keeps for at least a couple of weeks in the fridge, so make a large bottle full and enjoy.
When making a full bottle, substitute 4 tablesp. olive oil with 4 of herb flavored olive oil for a change of flavor.

Pesto

Serves 3-4

- a handful of fresh basil, chopped
- 2-3 tablesp. extra virgin olive oil
- sea salt – to taste
- 1 tablesp. pine nuts

1. Make the pesto by combining all ingredients and mixing well.

This will keep well in the fridge for a few days so you could make double or treble the amount and store in an air tight container.

Milk Substitutes

Double Cream

- 2 cups of sunflower oil (or rape seed oil or hemp oil)
- 1 cup of soya yoghurt
- 1/4 teaspoon liquid lecithin (can be soya or sunflower)
- 5 g of D ribose
- 1 teaspn. vanilla essence

1. Whizz up in a blender or a smoothie maker.

For really thick cream add a teaspoonful of linseed seed – these absorb any water and really thicken the cream!

Snacks and Goodies

Pork Scratchings

- Pork skin
- Salt

1. Buy pork skin, from a butcher's shop, with as much of the white fat removed as possible. (Sometimes the butcher's will give it away for free.)
2. Light oven 150C, Gas 3.
3. Cut the skin into inch wide strips and then cut into 3-4 inch lengths.
4. Place skin side up in a deep sided roasting tin.
5. Roast for 2 hours. Pour off the fat and replace the tin in the oven. Turn up the heat to Gas 8, 220C for 10-15 minutes till the skin is puffy and golden brown. Drain off any more fat and sprinkle with the salt to taste.
6. Cool. Then store in sealed freezer bags in the fridge and enjoy as a snack.

These only keep for a few days before the fat begins to taste rancid, so eat quickly and enjoy.

Tapenade

- 1 garlic clove, crushed
- 1 lemon, juice only
- 3 tablesp. capers, chopped
- 6 anchovy fillets, chopped
- 250g / 9oz black olives, pitted
- small bunch fresh parsley, chopped
- salt and freshly ground black pepper
- 2– 4 tablesp. extra virgin olive oil

1. To make a rough textured tapenade, simply mix all the ingredients together, adding enough olive oil to form a paste.
2. For a smoother texture, tip the garlic, lemon juice, capers and anchovy into a food processor and process for about 10 seconds.
3. Add the olives and parsley and process again with enough olive oil to make a paste.
4. Season to taste if necessary.

Tapenade can be served as an appetizer or a snack, spread on bread substitute.

Cinnamon Swirl Cake

To make the buttermilk:
- 1/4 cup water or soy, oat, almond milk
- 1 teasp Lemon Juice

Cake mix:
- 2 cups packed blanched almond flour
- 3/4 cup oat flour, tapioca flour or arrowroot
- 3/4 cup xylitol or truvia
- 1 teasp. baking powder (double acting if you have it!)
- 1/4 teasp. salt
- 1/3 cup melted coconut oil
- 2 large eggs
- 1 tables vanilla extract

Swirl Topping
- 1 tablesp cinnamon
- 1 1/2 tablesp xylitol or truvia dissolved in 1 tablesp hot water

1. Preheat oven to 350F, 180C, gas mark 4.
2. Line a small cake pan or bread pan with parchment paper.
3. In a small bowl combine the milk (or water) or your choice with the lemon juice. Set aside.
4. In a large bowl combine the almond flour, starch, sweetener, baking powder, salt and stir well. Add in the melted coconut oil, eggs, vanilla, milk (or water).
5. Scoop out 1/3 cup of the batter into a small bowl. To that batter add the cinnamon and sweetened syrup.
6. Pour the (white) batter into the parchment lined pan. Then drizzle the (brown) cinnamon batter over top in a marble like swirly pattern.
7. Place in oven. Bake for 40-45 minutes – a toothpick should come out clean. Let cool slightly before slicing.

Store at room temperature in a sealed container or freeze for another day!

Cinnamon Biscuits

Makes 9-10 large biscuits

- 2 packed cups blanched almond flour
- 1 teasp baking powder
- 1/4 teasp salt
- 1 teasp vanilla
- 2 tablesp milk of choice – soy, almond or oat
- 3 tablesp coconut oil
- 1/4 cup Truvia or xylitol
- 1 heaping teaspoon cinnamon

1. Preheat oven to 350f, 180C, gas 4 and line a baking sheet with parchment paper.
2. In a mixing bowl, combine the almond flour, baking powder, salt, vanilla, milk and butter.
3. In a separate bowl, mix the cinnamon and half of the stevia/xylitol together.
4. Pour the rest of the xylitol in the with dough and combine.
5. Roll the dough out into small balls and cover in the cinnamon mixture.
6. Flatten with the palm of your hand and line on the baking sheet.
7. This should make about 9-10 cookies.
8. Bake for 11-12 minutes.

Store in an air tight container.

Chocolate Coconut Squares

- 6 tablesp. coconut oil
- 4 tablesp. raw cacao powder
- Handful of cocoa nibs
- 1-2 teasp. xylitol according to taste
- 1 orange – use the zest and the juice
- 60-80g. Rude Health puffed oats
- 75 g. almonds and/or hazelnuts, roughly chopped.

1. Melt the coconut oil in a large bowl over a pan of hot water.
2. Add the raw cacao powder, the cocoa nibs, the xylitol, zest and juice of orange. Stir well.
3. When it's all thick but still runny add the nuts and enough puffed oats so that all the oats are covered with the chocolate mix.
4. Put into a non-stick Swiss roll tin or a greased shallow dish and press down well.
5. Allow to cool and set.
6. Cut into squares.
7. Place in an air tight container and keep in the fridge.

Drinks

Stone Age Coffee

Serves 1

- 1 tablesp. coconut oil
- 1 tablesp. hemp oil
- 1 tablesp. sunflower lecithin granules
- 1 tablesp. Vitalite butter or Pure spread
- 1 teasp. your favorite coffee
- Plus Xylitol or Stevia to sweeten if necessary
- Mug of hot water

1. Mix up fats and oils in a large mug.
2. Add coffee, sweeteners, lecithin granules.
Pour in about a 3 of the mug with water so when you use a hand blender for 30secs it doesn't spill. Blend till white and frothy like milky coffee.
3. Top up with more hot water and stir!
4. Drink hot.

Bedtime Cocoa

Serves 1

- 1 tablesp. coconut oil
- 1 tablesp. hemp oil
- 1 tablesp. sunflower lecithin
- 1 teasp. green & black cocoa powder
- Xylitol or stevia to sweeten
- soya milk or kefir

1. Place oils, Lecithin and cocoa powder in large mug. Top up with hot water and stir well.
2. Add soy, almond milk or kefir to taste and stir well. Drink while hot.

Stone Age Anytime Cuppasoup

Serves 1

- 1 tablesp. hemp oil
- 1 tablesp. sunflower lecithin granules
- 1 tablesp. coconut oil
- 1 tablesp. Marigold Swiss bouillon

1. Mix all ingredients to a paste in a large mug.
2. Add hot water.
3. Stir well.

Drink hot.

Made in the USA
Middletown, DE
10 July 2021